'Every home should have a copy of this book which provides practical tips about how to receive the best health care. *Ten Questions You Must Ask Your Doctor* is a well-researched book that explores how and why modern medicine is letting us down. Health professionals, particularly those in training, should study the examples in this book so they can begin to prepare their answers.'

Professor Rachelle Buchbinder
Monash University, Melbourne

'Doctors usually put the interests of their patients first, but they nevertheless sometimes do them more harm than good. This may be because they haven't kept up-to-date with trustworthy research evidence, and sometimes because their practice has been unduly influenced by commercial considerations. Melissa Sweet's and Ray Moynihan's book will help patients to be aware of these problems and to work with their physicians to reduce them.'

Sir Iain Chalmers
James Lind Library, Oxford

Other books by Ray Moynihan and Melissa Sweet

Ray Moynihan, *Too Much Medicine?*
Ray Moynihan and Alan Cassels, *Selling Sickness: How drug companies are turning us all into patients*
Melissa Sweet, *The Big Fat Conspiracy: How to protect your family's health*
Melissa Sweet with Les Irwig, Judy Irwig, and Lyndal Trevena, *Smart Health Choices*, editions 1 and 2
Melissa Sweet, *Inside Madness*

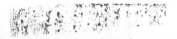

HOW PATIENTS SHOULD THINK

10 QUESTIONS TO ASK
YOUR DOCTOR ABOUT
DRUGS, TESTS, AND TREATMENT

RAY MOYNIHAN
& MELISSA SWEET

PEGASUS BOOKS
NEW YORK

HOW PATIENTS SHOULD THINK

Pegasus Books LLC
80 Broad Street
5th Floor
New York, NY 10004

Library of Congress Cataloging-in-Publication Data is available.

ISBN: 978-1-60598-047-8

10 9 8 7 6 5 4 3 2 1

Printed in the United States of America
Distributed by W. W. Norton & Company, Inc.
www.pegasusbooks.us

Contents

Foreword

Good health is something we all prize more than most things in life. It is sometimes hard to put a value on it, but we certainly know what it means when we do not have it. Keeping well has to be a partnership between us and our health providers— each has a responsibility in that relationship—and that relationship has to be built on trust and communication.

Ray Moynihan and Melissa Sweet have a reputation for asking the hard questions about health and the health system, and have now written this book on what we should be asking health practitioners about our health and suggested treatments. Patient involvement in clinical decision making is so important. No longer do we want to be told about the condition we have (or think we have), what it might lead to and the various treatment options without a clear explanation. More and more, we want to be involved in those decisions, but we need information so we can make reasonably informed decisions.

The health care system itself is very complex and navigating through it needs careful planning. It is not easy to know where or to whom we should go for a particular health problem. Each of us should have a good general practitioner who we can trust and with whom we, and other members of the health care team, can work through our particular health problem.

It is important to understand there are often a number of different ways of tackling the same problem—including surgery, medicines, even physical exercise. What is important is that we feel we have been able to get information we can use effectively—and trust.

Ten Questions You Must Ask Your Doctor is the book to help us navigate complex health systems which, I think, are often designed for the health professionals and the health industry rather than patients. Ray Moynihan and Melissa Sweet, who have a reputation for getting to the truth, guide us to make informed health decisions and give us the questions we need to ask: what have I got, what investigations should I have done, what are the options about surgery or medicines, and what can I do to prevent this happening again? They raise important questions regarding how we might think about information provided, particularly from the media or that produced by the health industry. They also discuss issues of the conflict of interest that can arise from the interaction between health professionals and the health industry. Dwight Eisenhower, a Republican president of the United States, often talked about his concern with the military–industrial complex—the links between armaments manufacturers and nation states who might discourage peace as this would influence sales of their wares. We should now be aware of the power of the medical–industrial complex and realise that although it is a force for good and that incredible advances in medicine have been made—sometimes it may favour profit (and there is nothing wrong with profit) over the interests of patients.

Communication is a two way process. It has to be remembered that many health practitioners are still coming to terms with the informed patient and feel very uneasy about being questioned by them. This book will help that dialogue by providing a clear list of the things we should be asking of our health provider—and not just when we have a health problem. It underlines the responsibility we have to understand (love) and look after our bodies. This is so important because we have to place increasing emphasis on health rather than sickness as we move through the new millennium. We cannot just fund or support what is effectively an 'illth' system. We currently spend less than 10 per cent of our health budget on disease prevention and health promotion and 90 per cent on acute care and the hospital system. If we are going to cope with the ageing population and with chronic disease, it is becoming increasingly important that we take more responsibility for our own health, what we eat, how much we exercise and develop a relationship with our health advisors so that our interactions with the health system are kept to a minimum.

Professor Peter Brooks
Executive Dean, Health Sciences, University of Queensland

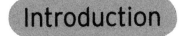

Introduction

Why you need to ask your doctor some tough questions

Our health is one of the most precious things we have. Yet our health *system* can put our health at risk. Too often we receive tests, treatments, pills and procedures that are useless, unnecessary and even harmful.[1] This book will help you and your loved ones avoid such unhelpful care by bringing a more questioning approach to your dealings with doctors and other health professionals.

The great advances of high-tech medicine have saved millions of lives, but they have also created some unhealthy myths. Many of us believe that everything our doctors do has been scientifically tested, that health professionals always have our best interests at heart, and that hospitals and clinics are safe places devoted to helping patients. The reality is that many common therapies are very poorly tested, health professionals sometimes act out of self-interest, and profit-driven medical corporations are performing tests and procedures that patients may not actually need.

We, the authors, are two journalists who specialise in covering health and medical issues. Between us, we have many years experience with leading newspapers and magazines, television and radio stations, medical journals and universities, in Australia, North America and Europe. And like anyone else, we have had our own personal experiences of the health system. For both of us, serious illness has touched our lives and the lives of our families and close friends. We are intimately aware of the best and worst of medicine and health care.

Asking questions of doctors and other health professionals is also our business. As a result of asking these questions, there has been a fundamental shift in the way we view health care. The more you learn about modern health care, the more likely you are to end up with a healthy scepticism about its potential benefits and harms. You begin to appreciate that the picture is far less rosy and far more complicated than that promoted by the TV medical dramas. There is often enormous controversy and conflict within the medical profession over what works, how well it works, and who exactly should be receiving treatment. With this book, we want to share some of what we have learnt through our combined years of health reporting.

One of the most damaging myths of all is that the more health care you get, the healthier you'll be. The truth is that many of us are getting far 'too much of a good thing'. Along with their potential benefits, all treatments carry potential harms, and things can go wrong even when a procedure is necessary. Most of us do not appreciate just how many uncertainties and risks surround modern health care.

The good news is that there is a growing amount of reliable information to help us all make better decisions. Many health systems around the world are undergoing radical change, with the aim of making everyone more aware of the pros and cons of different treatments, the benefits and the risks. Power, which traditionally lay in the hands of doctors and other health professionals, is starting to be shared more fairly. People everywhere are being encouraged and supported to become more informed about their health care and to have a greater say in the decisions that affect their health and well-being. No longer is it assumed that we should simply 'follow doctor's orders'. A perfect example of this change is the development of 'decision aids', which give patients balanced information about their options. They are available for common conditions such as breast and prostate cancer, to help patients weigh up the potential benefits and harms of different tests and treatments.

The success of this revolution in health care depends on us being more willing and able to speak up and ask questions. That means we need to know what questions to ask, why we're asking them, and then make sense of the answers. And if you don't get those questions answered in a way you can understand, you have to know how to find other trustworthy sources of health information that can help. *Ten Questions You Must Ask Your Doctor* will help you do just that: it will help you to ask the questions that could make a huge difference to your health and well-being, and to understand what the answers mean in your situation.

The book is based around ten key questions that anyone interacting with health services and health professionals of any type should understand, whether the dealings are with doctors, dentists, naturopaths, nurses, chiropractors, acupuncturists or physiotherapists. The structure is broken into three sections: questions about tests, questions about treatments, and some general questions. Each question is the basis of a chapter and each chapter uses three common examples to demonstrate why asking that particular question is so important.

One such example is back pain, a widespread ailment. So, for instance, the chapter encouraging you to ask 'What are my options?' examines how people with back pain may end up having unnecessary tests and potentially harmful treatments if they don't get this question fully answered *before* making decisions about their back. As you will read, the safest option for many people with back pain may well be to avoid invasive tests and treatments altogether. As with so many other common complaints, Mother Nature, if given the time and opportunity, is often the best healer. Sometimes, as the saying goes, less is more. Or, to put it another way, the less medical intervention, the better. And sometimes, of course, powerful drugs or major surgery are needed, and can be life-saving.

In this book, we have tended to choose examples that highlight the use of tests and treatments that may not work or are even harmful. Many people may not realise how widespread this problem is. However, there are also many examples—not covered in this book—of peole missing out on tests and treatments of proven benefit. The powerful health and medical industry devotes much effort to addressing the issue of under-treatment, although usually only where there's a market. We seek to get a more healthy balance in the public debate by drawing attention to the other side of the equation—in order to reduce the suffering and waste caused by unnecessary interventions.

There is no need to read the chapters in the order they appear. You may be more interested in some than others. This is not a book you need to read cover to cover, but it is a book you will want to talk about with friends, loved ones and those who provide your health care.

Even though asking questions is our business, we admit that we too can find it difficult to do this when visiting doctors as patients ourselves or when supporting family members or friends. If you're sick and in an unfamiliar environment, like a hospital or doctor's surgery, and you know the doctor is rushed and has a waiting room full of patients, the thought of asking a lot of questions can be very intimidating.

Asking questions can be daunting enough, but sometimes the answers can be frightening too. The more you ask, the more you will learn, and sometimes that means more complexity and uncertainty. Some people might prefer to stay in the dark and keep things simple. Increasingly, however, many of us want to know as much as we can, and be as informed as possible before we make major decisions.

In writing the book, we do not imagine that you would ask all of the ten questions whenever you see a doctor. You may, however, find that one or two are relevant to your situation at any given consultation. Our aim is to try to encourage a questioning approach, because the more questions you ask, the more quickly you will learn how to avoid useless and dangerous treatments and discover what's safe and effective. Our hope is that the way you think about your health and health care may start to change if you consider the ten chapters that follow. And we hope it will empower you to become sceptical and questioning about health advice generally.

For the sake of convenience, we often refer to 'doctors' throughout this book, but the questions we raise are relevant for any source of health advice, whether a doctor, dentist, naturopath, newspaper article, website, neighbour or friend. Similarly, we refer to 'tests' and 'treatments' as a way of encompassing the full range of health and medical interventions on offer, whether vitamin pills, X-rays or surgical procedures.

This book is not only for people who are ill or seeking advice from health professionals. It is for anyone interested in finding out what they can do themselves to benefit their well-being. Every day, we all make decisions that affect our health. It might be what we choose to eat, whether we drive or walk to the shops, or deciding whether to have another glass of wine or beer. Preserving our precious health means much more than simply asking questions of our doctor or other health professional. It also means asking questions about what we can do for our own well-being.

The choices and decisions you make can affect your chances of staying healthy or, if you are unwell, maximise your chances of recovery or simply managing your condition. In every sense, this book aims to give you greater control over your health and health care.

QUESTIONS ABOUT YOUR DIAGNOSIS

One

Do I really need that test?

X-rays, blood tests and high-tech scans can be life-saving. Medical tests are extremely valuable tools for diagnosing diseases, and then guiding decisions about what treatments might help. Testing of patients is becoming more and more common in doctors' surgeries, hospitals, dentists' rooms and other places where health services are delivered. The problem is that many of these tests are unnecessary.

An unnecessary test is not just a waste of your time and money: it can also be a threat to your health. Tests often appear to be simple and harmless, but this is rarely the case, as we will see from the three common examples discussed in this chapter.

Tests themselves can have serious side effects and sometimes even cause deadly disease. In some cases, having one test can lead you to a whole lot more tests and treatments that may in the end do you more harm than good. And, finally, having a test can be the first step towards making an otherwise healthy person feel as if they're sick.

'Do I really need that test?' is a question that should be asked much more often, even when the test seems quick and painless.

One morning, a couple of years ago, Steven Birnbaum received one of those phone calls that parents fear most. His 23-year-old daughter Molly had been hit by a car while jogging and rushed to a nearby hospital. When Steven arrived at intensive care, his daughter was conscious but had serious head injuries. Thanks to the wonders of modern testing technology, the doctors had worked out that Molly's main injuries were a fractured skull and severe concussion, but she was likely to make a full recovery. They knew this because Molly had undergone a sophisticated type of X-ray known as a computerised tomography, or CT scan. As she lay on an examination table which slowly slid her body into the big CT machine, multiple X-rays were taken, giving doctors a clear view of the inside of her head.[1]

Molly's dad, Steven Birnbaum, was able to make sense of the results of her CT scans and confirm that the treating doctors had got her diagnosis right. That's because Steven himself was a radiologist, a specialist doctor who works with CT scans and other tests like X-rays every day.

As radiologists like Steven know all too well, modern tests regularly save lives. Blood tests detect deadly viruses like HIV/AIDS, X-rays reveal broken bones and ultrasounds can show up suspect internal lumps. Old-fashioned methods of diagnosing illness, like doctors taking a detailed history from the patient, remain as valuable as ever, yet few people would argue with the notion that sophisticated modern tests have helped many patients. And apart from helping find disease, having a medical test is also often a way of reassuring us that we are free of illness, and nothing is wrong. A normal test result can provide great relief.

The problem, of course, is too much of a good thing. In recent decades the use of tests in medicine has skyrocketed. In 1980 in the United States there were 3 million CT scans conducted. Now there are **Too many tests can mean too much of a good thing** more than 60 million every year.[2] That's a twentyfold increase. In Australia there has been similar rapid growth in the use of tests, which has caused serious financial headaches for those running the national health system, Medicare. The massive increases have been driven by many factors. Some doctors fear being sued, so they order tests to cover themselves rather than believing they are really necessary for their patient's welfare. Sometimes patients ask for a test they don't really need, without understanding the full consequences. And very importantly, many companies and individuals profit handsomely from the sale and use of tests.

More and more people around the world are becoming concerned about the overuse of tests. Increasingly, they are saying 'enough is enough'. Dr Steven Birnbaum is one of them.

Back in intensive care, on the morning of Molly's second day in hospital, Steven was still at his daughter's bedside. On the first day the treating doctors had ordered several scans, all of which Steven thought were appropriate and necessary to make a quick diagnosis of what was wrong. But by the second day, he was becoming concerned. After Molly's doctors had ordered three more CT scans, her father decided 'no more'. He felt the tests being ordered were unwarranted. Like any type of X-ray, CT scans expose the body to radiation, and Steven feared that his daughter was being exposed unnecessarily to potentially dangerous levels of radiation.

As a radiologist himself, working in the United States, Steven Birnbaum was becoming more and more worried by the number of scans being performed at the hospitals where he worked. He feared that too many people were being exposed to too much radiation, and he was horrified that it was happening to his own daughter. He asked one of the people in charge of her care whether they had given any thought to what radiation levels they were exposing patients to in their hospital. They hadn't. Steven was incensed. Like many others around the world, he is now working to make us all more aware of the dangers of these seemingly innocent scans.

Despite the enormous increase in the numbers of tests being performed in recent years, there is no good evidence that that increase has led to a similar increase in our health as a population. Major studies in the United States, where unwanted testing is the most out of control, show that in some parts of the country, three times more tests are given per capita than elsewhere. This has not meant that people from highly tested areas have better health.[3] The concern is that an awful lot of money is being wasted, and an awful lot of people are having tests they do not need. It is now time to start routinely asking your doctor, dentist, acupuncturist or physiotherapist whether you really do need that test.

While medical tests might seem simple and harmless, they are not. There are three possible downsides that may have to be weighed up before you take a test. First, tests themselves can

Tests are not simple or harmless

cause physical and psychological side effects, like infection or anxiety. Second, tests can give unreliable results, perhaps suggesting that you need treatment when you may not. And finally, having a simple, common test might mean you end up being labelled as having a disease or dysfunction that you may have to live with for the rest of your life. Sometimes such a label can help open doors to valuable treatments like effective drugs, but other times we can end up being labelled as sick and suffering from any number of new disorders, when we may in fact be in reasonably good health. For all these reasons it is worth thinking very seriously before having any tests done, asking whether they really need to be done, and whether there might be some better alternatives.

The aim is not to avoid tests altogether, because so many of them can be helpful. The aim instead is to try to avoid the ones that are not needed. But whether a particular scan or blood test is necessary, is not always clear. Different people will react differently to the same information about the benefits and downsides of having any given test. The point is to try to get as much information as possible to help you make the most informed decision. While we all have a natural curiosity and often want to know all we can about what might be wrong with us or our loved ones, having a test can sometimes lead us down potentially rocky pathways we never really needed to step onto.

Tests themselves can cause serious harm. As the example on CT scans in this chapter shows, common tests that use radiation—like X-rays and CT scans—are strongly suspected of causing cancer. It is very shocking to learn that you only need to have a small number of these scans before you start to raise your risk of cancer. Unbelievably, the common X-ray has recently been classified as cancer-causing and labelled as a 'carcinogen' by the World Health Organization.[4]

Tests can start us down a pathway to more tests

Apart from physical harm, there is also the psychological anxiety that can arise when you get a test. As many of us know, waiting for the results of a test for serious illness can be agonising.[5] Even if the results come back normal, many people are understandably still not reassured and continue to worry for a long time afterwards.[6] But if the test wasn't warranted in the first place, all that worry has happened unnecessarily. The whole process of testing can be much more onerous than we imagine.

Tests can start us down a pathway to more tests and then to potentially risky or unproven treatments. In the second example on the PSA blood test, which is widely used to help diagnose prostate cancer in men, we see that even commonly used tests can be unreliable. Many test results are not black and white, but rather very uncertain in terms of what they actually mean, despite the fact that doctors often appear certain when they tell you about them. And unreliable tests can sometimes lead to a false diagnosis—or an all-clear that is unwarranted. You can't rely on doctors or other health professionals to automatically tell you about the uncertainties surrounding many tests; often it's up to you to ask questions like: 'Do I really need this test?'

Even the simplest of tests can produce results that will change our lives forever. The third example in this chapter examines a blood test for cholesterol levels and highlights how having a test can result in a medical label that you may wear for the rest of your life. Sometimes receiving a correct diagnosis and a label is absolutely necessary, because it can lead to valuable treatments. But sometimes that label might actually be unhelpful, because it can cause people to think of themselves as sick or diseased when they are in reality healthy.

Tests can produce results that will change our lives forever

EXAMPLE 1
CT scanning

The reason radiologist Steven Birnbaum was so concerned about his daughter receiving too many CT scans is that they involve large doses of radiation. Computerised tomography scans are used all over the body, from the head and chest to the stomach and heart. Unlike ultrasounds or MRIs, which use different methods of seeing inside the body, CT scans, X-rays and nuclear medicine tests all use radiation. One CT scan can give a dose of roughly 10 units of radiation (a unit here is referring to a millisievert, or mSv). Yet just 50 units of radiation, the amount received from five CT scans, may lead to an increased risk of cancer later in life.[7]

Tests themselves can cause harm

Much of the evidence about cancer risk comes from studies of survivors of the nuclear bomb explosions in the Japanese cities of Hiroshima and Nagasaki, who were exposed to radiation at the end of the Second World War. More research on this is needed because exactly what dose of radiation will increase your risk of cancer, and by how much, is still uncertain. The point here is not to cause alarm about the CT scans or other tests that you or your loved ones may have had in the past. Rather the aim is to encourage scepticism regarding the tests that you might be recommended in the future.[8]

For many years there have been concerns about the radiation people are exposed to when they receive X-rays and CT scans, but now mainstream medical associations are taking the issue very seriously indeed. In 2007, the conservative American College of Radiology released an alarming paper on the potential dangers of radiation, produced by a special panel which included Dr Steven Birnbaum.[9] Because of the massive increase in the number of tests being done, the paper described a 'significant increase in the population's cumulative exposure to ionizing radiation'. Will this lead to an increase in the rates of cancer? The paper was uncertain but stated, 'the presumption is that it will'.

As that document outlines, there is still uncertainty about how serious these dangers are, and there is an urgent need to start doing more research to find out what harm these scans are doing to people. There are ongoing doubts about what doses of radiation many machines give out, and about how much radiation is absorbed into different parts of the human body. The document also states that many doctors who order tests for their patients do not even think about the dose of radiation that their patients will receive. While some doctors are very knowledgeable, it says that others 'have had little or no training in radiation exposure and do not routinely consider this factor when ordering imaging examinations'. The report urges radiologists themselves to be more open with their patients about the potential cancer risks of tests like CT scans.

As anyone who has had a scan recently would know, trying to meet and talk with the radiologist who reads your scan result is almost impossible, let alone ask them questions. Tough questions really need to be put to the doctor, physiotherapist or chiropractor who is referring you for a CT scan, for example: 'Do I really need this test?' and 'Does the test itself involve any potential harms or side effects?' These questions are even more important when a health professional recommends that a child be scanned and exposed to radiation. The dose of radiation that children receive from CT scans can vary enormously, and there are growing concerns that too many children are receiving too many scans, exposing them to too much radiation.[10]

Significant concerns about too much radiation are the potential long-term damage to a child's development and the increased risk of cancer.[11] In 2006, a Canadian auditor-general heavily criticised hospitals in one province after discovering an excessive use of CT scans on kids.[12] Problems included hospitals not using special settings for smaller bodies, and failing to monitor the size of the doses and the number of scans children received. The auditor-general's report also referred to a survey of Canadian doctors, revealing that over 90 per cent of them underestimated the radiation dose that children received from a CT scan.

While there are moves underway to try to reduce the number of CT scans and the amount of radiation that children and adults are exposed to, these scans remain big business. Doctors, private hospital companies and medical centres will not give up precious profits without a fight. In the United States, X-rays and CT and other scans are called 'diagnostic imaging tests'—and when you add them all up, they make a US$100 billion a year industry.[13] Many individual doctors own the testing machines they have in their surgeries, which means they benefit directly whenever they recommend that test to a patient. There is very good evidence to show that when a doctor has a financial interest in ordering a test, they will order a lot more of them. Normally such behaviour would be seen as something like an illegal 'kickback' but, under a special exemption in the law, doctors are allowed to do it.[14]

Similarly, in Australia, the large companies that own local medical centres may also own testing equipment and pathology laboratories. That means there is a financial incentive for the medical centre owners to encourage their doctors to send patients for tests, as we will hear more about in chapter 9, 'Who else is profiting?'.

In recent years, many specialist radiologists in Australia have formed themselves into highly profitable companies, which have invested heavily in million-dollar machinery like CT scanners. These doctors have an obvious interest in earning profits from those machines, which means having the maximum number of people come through the door every day for a test. There is a lot of pressure out there in some sectors of the medical marketplace to take a CT scan, and growing evidence that too many of us may be having them. In fact, a recent study in Australia suggested that perhaps two-thirds of all CT scans of the chest may be inappropriate.[15] One way to protect against unnecessary and potentially dangerous scans for you or your children is to ask beforehand very firmly: 'Do I really need this test?'

EXAMPLE 2
PSA testing

A PSA (or prostate-specific antigen) blood test is one of the most common medical tests given to men in many parts of the world. It's also one of the most controversial. If ever there was a time to ask 'Do I really need this test?', it's when your doctor suggests a PSA test to check for prostate cancer. It's doubly important to ask this when the test is ordered as part of a general check-up, without it even being specifically discussed with the patient. The decision to have a test rests with the individual. However, it is worth knowing that there are many people who have looked closely at the pros and cons of this and believe that far too many men are being given the PSA test unnecessarily.

Unreliable tests can lead to unproven treatments

Part of the problem is that the PSA blood test is not designed to detect prostate cancer directly. It actually measures prostate-specific antigen, a protein in the blood which is produced by the prostate, the small gland that sits below a man's bladder. PSA levels in the blood can be high because of a number of factors, including cancer, but also the very common and less serious problem of having an enlarged or inflamed prostate. This means that the results of a PSA test are often not very clear. A PSA test alone does not give doctors enough information to distinguish between benign prostate conditions and the potentially more serious cancer, and so more tests, including biopsies, will often follow.

The danger here is that what appears to be a simple blood test can in fact be the beginning of a complicated chain of procedures that can eventually cause side effects, and which may turn out to have been totally unnecessary in the first place. As two American researchers put it recently, the PSA test can lead to a 'cascade of unanticipated events'.[16] We need to know before any test is done exactly what those 'unanticipated events' might be. If your general practitioner or specialist can't answer your questions and refer you to reliable information so you can learn more, then they shouldn't be recommending the test.

A key problem with many medical tests is that they can sometimes give the wrong answer. In other words, the results might suggest that you may have a disease when you don't. That's called a 'false positive' result. On the other hand, test results can suggest that you don't have a disease, when in fact you may. That's called a 'false negative' result. The PSA test is a good example of a test that can produce a lot of both false positive and false negative results.

Sometimes the PSA test result will come up all clear, when in fact the man has prostate cancer; there are estimates this kind of 'false negative' result can happen about 15 per cent of the time with this test. On the other hand, the results may suggest a man might have cancer, and following further tests he will find that he doesn't; estimates find that this kind of 'false positive' happens more than 50 per cent of the time with the PSA test.[17]

One obvious problem with a false positive result from a PSA test is that men will be subjecting themselves to further tests that might themselves carry complications. For instance, a biopsy may be recommended to check whether the cancer is there, which involves removing small pieces of living tissue from the prostate gland—sometimes many small pieces of tissue. This procedure can cause pain, infection and bleeding. And some men who receive a 'false positive' result may also be caused to worry a lot unnecessarily.

Researchers recently compared the anxiety levels of two groups of men who had had the PSA test. One group of men had 'negative' test results suggesting they were normal and free from cancer. The other group had a 'false positive': they had an abnormal result to their PSA test but later found out, after having a biopsy, that they didn't have cancer. The researchers discovered that more men who received a 'false positive' result thought and worried about cancer, compared to those whose tests results were initially negative.[18] This is not surprising, but it does remind us that being told you might have cancer, when you don't, can have a major psychological impact, and that it is important to ask up-front whether the test is warranted in the first place.

Perhaps the biggest problem with the PSA test is this: even if further tests show the presence of cancer, there is great uncertainty about the best way to treat it, whether some men should be treated at all, and whether for some men the cancer is best left untreated.[19] Prostate cancer can be very slow-growing, and while a large percentage of all older men have the cancer in their bodies, only a very small percentage ever die from it. One recent estimate suggested that less than 1 per cent of men in their sixties will die from prostate cancer in the coming decade.[20] That's why one of the commonly recommended ways of treating this cancer is called 'watchful waiting', which basically means getting no treatment unless there are signs the cancer is growing and posing a threat to health. The other treatment options include radical surgery, which can carry serious side effects including impotence and a very small risk of death (see chapter 3, 'Do I really need to be screened?', for more). Examining all the evidence, many doctors and health authorities around the world believe that routinely testing healthy men with a PSA test is inappropriate.[21]

The main point here is not to warn men against getting a PSA test. The aim is to encourage men and their families to ask questions and consider all the implications of having such a test, as well as encouraging a healthy scepticism towards all tests. Many tests can appear simple and harmless but could be the beginning of a very difficult, and potentially unwarranted, chain of events.

EXAMPLE 3
Cholesterol tests

Cholesterol tests are so common these days, and fears about high cholesterol so deeply embedded in our culture, that it seems sacrilegious to even question the need for these tests. **A quick test can lead to a lifelong medical label** But like other very common tests for high blood pressure or thinning bones, it is worth thinking a bit about what the consequences of a cholesterol test might be, before having it.

One of the important consequences is that you may end up with a lifelong label. Someone who has 'high cholesterol' is often portrayed as someone suffering from a serious medical condition, when in fact high cholesterol is really only one risk factor for future heart attack or stroke—others include smoking, physical inactivity and poor diet.

Rather than being some deadly substance, cholesterol is an essential compound in the human body. For people at high risk of heart attack or stroke, having high levels of cholesterol can be a bad thing according to current medical wisdom, and lowering it may lower those risks. But for others at lower risk of heart disease to begin with, the picture is a lot less certain. For many people, a lot can be done to lower risks of heart attack by quitting smoking, reducing drinking, eating and exercising better—without ever needing to turn your problem into a medical one. Taking a cholesterol test and becoming a life-long 'patient' as a result may not always be the best thing to do. Indeed, a small number of people who have looked at all the research on 'high cholesterol' suggest it may not play a significant role at all in producing heart disease, though that view is highly controversial.[22]

Weighed against that controversial view is very strong evidence that if you are a person at high risk of heart disease, long-term use of cholesterol-lowering drugs can decrease the risk of heart attacks and other illnesses. Let's take a hypothetical case. A middle-aged person facing a two in ten chance of a potentially deadly heart attack may be able to reduce that chance to one in ten if they take cholesterol-lowering drugs for several years. Or put another way, for every ten such people prescribed these drugs, one will have a heart attack prevented. Certainly don't take those figures as being relevant to you, but they do provide a sense of how effective the drugs can be for some people at high risk. For other people at lower risk to begin with, the benefits of drugs are much less pronounced.

As you probably know, one of the very likely results of being positively tested for high cholesterol is that your doctor will recommend treatment with cholesterol-lowering drugs like Lipitor, which is one of the most heavily marketed medicines of all time. Again, if you have already had a heart attack or stroke, or if you have a strong family history of heart disease or stroke, the drugs may reduce your risk in a meaningful way. But if you are reasonably healthy and at fairly low risk of future heart attack, taking these drugs long term could be costly, wasteful and potentially dangerous. While cholesterol drugs are regarded as being generally free of side effects, for some of them there are very serious, though very rare, complications—including wasting away of the muscles, which can be life-threatening.[23]

Another aspect to consider is that too much focus on high cholesterol, and the drugs that lower it, can distract attention from all the other strategies that will lower your risk of heart attack and stroke, namely changes to diet and lifestyle. If you are in reasonable health, you need to ask questions about whether a cholesterol test is going to lead you down a path towards lifelong drug-taking which may do you more harm than good.

Conclusion

Do I really need that test?

Steven Birnbaum's daughter Molly has recovered well from the injuries sustained in her accident. But the excessive number of CT scans that were ordered for her in hospital inspired her father afterwards to become a self-described 'zealot', warning the world about the dangers of 'too much of a good thing', which was the title of an article he published recently in a leading medical journal.[24] Many doctors and other health professionals will be resistant to anyone questioning their authority to recommend tests and scans. Yet the evidence that some tests are wasteful and harmful is abundant and clear. The sad reality of profit-driven medicine is that when a doctor orders a test for you, it may be that others gain a lot more from it than you do.

You may not always have the opportunity to ask questions about the tests being ordered—if it's an emergency, for example. But when there is time, asking some important questions about tests—like the ones opposite—might in the long run save you time and money, as well as being good for your health.

More questions about tests

Do I really need that test?

- What will the results mean?
- What are the chances of the test finding disease when there isn't any?
- Does the test itself involve any potential harms or side effects?
- What are the possible treatments if the test is positive?
- What will all this cost?
- Are there other testing options that are more reliable and less dangerous?

Two

Do I really have that disorder?

Many healthy people are wrongly told they are sick. If you or a loved one is told you have an illness or a disorder, there are good reasons to question whether or not this is actually the case. The definitions of 'old' illnesses are being widened all the time, and 'new' conditions are being created.

Pharmaceutical company marketing strategies are helping to broaden the definitions of diseases in order to expand markets for their products. Sometimes these definitions are being expanded so much that they are catching lots of healthy people in the net. The danger is that by accepting an unwarranted medical label, you or your loved ones may end up receiving unnecessary tests and treatments that waste money and cause harm.

Just a little older than a toddler, the young preschooler looked shyly around the surgery. His mother and her doctor were discussing whether or not the boy had attention deficit hyperactivity disorder (ADHD), and whether he should be put on powerful drugs to treat it. One of the mum's other sons, just a year or two older than his little brother, had already been diagnosed with ADHD and was taking stimulant medications. After a not-too-lengthy consultation, the doctor decided the younger son also had the disorder, so he wrote a prescription and sent the family on its way.

The preschooler was old enough to talk, but he was not quite old enough to ask for himself, 'Do I really have that disorder?' It's a question his mother should have asked the doctor on her son's behalf. Particularly because that same doctor would reveal confidentially to one of the authors of this book, just a short time after that consultation, that he really wasn't even sure whether the boy had the disorder at all.[1]

One in ten young boys in the United States has been told he has ADHD and is being medicated with amphetamines and other stimulant drugs to treat it.[2] Similarly, in some parts of Australia, ADHD drugs are now extremely common-place in the classroom. While some children at the severe end of the spectrum may benefit from being diagnosed and taking prescription drugs, there is a widespread view that too many 'normal' kids are being told they have a disorder when they don't. The controversy about this disorder is fairly well-known, but ADHD is really just one example of a much bigger problem: too many people are told they have dysfunctions, diseases and disorders when they don't.[3]

Protecting yourself and your loved ones from an unnecessary medical label may end up being very good for your health.

Ordinary life is portrayed as medical disease

Sometimes there is no doubt about what's wrong and no real need to ask awkward questions about whether or not a doctor's diagnosis is correct. A badly broken leg is pretty clearly a badly broken leg. But as the medical profession and health care industries have grown in recent years, so too have the number of illnesses which you might be told you suffer from. As doctors and drug companies seek to expand the numbers of people they can treat and sell drugs to, more and more aspects of ordinary life are being classified as medical disease. This is not a conspiracy; it's just the way the medical marketplace works these days, particularly when the profit motive increasingly dominates within health care, as it does most visibly in the United States.

The definitions of diseases are often not set in stone, but rather they are elastic, and changing all the time. They are, however, changing in one direction—they are expanding. While it might seem as if these definitions are unable to be questioned, this is simply not true. Diseases are defined by small groups of men and women sitting in rooms working on computers like everyone else. And like everyone else, these people have biases and blind spots. The more you learn about the world of medicine, the more you realise that there is a lot of controversy surrounding the definition of disease, and it is often very unclear as to who should be defined as being sick. It's an amazing fact that exactly the same person with the same ailment might be described as perfectly healthy in one country, but sick in another.

There has always been a sense that cultural attitudes affect what we think of as illness. It wasn't so long ago that homosexuality and the menopause were portrayed as diseases. But over the last few decades, culture has started taking a back seat to commerce as drug companies and doctors realise you can make a lot of money telling healthy people they are sick.

When you take a close look at the definitions of many common diseases, and how they are changing over time, you are struck by the fact that in many cases the definitions just keep getting broader and broader, with more and more people being defined as ill. Attention Deficit Hyperactivity Disorder is a perfect example of this phenomenon, and the first example we deal with in this chapter. In the last thirty years there have been at least three changes to the definition of this disorder, which is slowly widening and catching greater numbers of kids—and now adults too—in the net. The more people defined as sick, the busier the doctor's surgery and the bigger the sales of the cures.

Being at risk of having a disease is not the same as having a disease. And yet increasingly the health and medical industries are acting as if these are the same thing. It's another reason to be sceptical when you are diagnosed with a disease. Having high cholesterol or high blood pressure doesn't mean you have a disease, it means you may be at increased risk of having an illness down the track.

A very good example here is osteoporosis, which is now commonly described as a 'silent killer' disease. In fact, osteoporosis is the loss of bony tissue that tends to happen as we age, which can modestly increase the risk that we might experience fractures. The real health problem is trying to prevent fractures, and there are many ways to do that without having to tell millions of healthy people they are suffering from a lifelong disease. Because drug companies have seen huge markets among older women for osteoporosis drugs, they have pumped tens of millions of dollars into public awareness campaigns over many years, helping to create widespread fears of this so-called disease. In fact, one group of respected researchers in Canada, who looked closely at the way osteoporosis was being sold to the public, described the selling of this condition as 'The Marketing of Fear'.[4]

Sometimes whole new diseases are created, as is happening now with a condition described as 'female sexual dysfunction'.[5] It is obvious to anyone that many people—men and women—experience sexual difficulties. These are extremely common. But over the last decade or so, a group of doctors and researchers, often working with drug company money, have defined what they describe as a new 'dysfunction', which they claim affects 43 per cent of all women. Most of the major 'scientific' meetings where this 'dysfunction' has been debated and defined have been heavily sponsored by drug companies, who are looking forward to the creation of giant new markets for their drugs. As we will learn in the third example in this chapter, a lot of people are challenging the creation of this condition. Before you accept any diagnosis of 'female sexual dysfunction', you may want to ask your doctor very confidently: 'Do I really have that disorder?'

The downsides of being diagnosed with an illness you don't have are pretty clear, but they are worth reminding ourselves about just the same. Walking around with a lifelong label—thinking you suffer from an illness when you don't—can cause an awful lot of wasted anxiety. The other key problem, of course, is that after being tested for a disease and accepting a medical label, you expose yourself to more tests and treatments which can involve serious side effects. As we will see, for example, the side effects from drugs for ADHD and osteoporosis can be harmful. And finally, there is a real waste of resources when people with mild problems are diagnosed and treated. Given the amount of genuine serious illness in the world, and the number of people suffering from painful and life-threatening disease, it seems absurd and unfair to waste resources treating those who are relatively healthy.

EXAMPLE 1
ADHD

If someone suggests that you or your child may have attention deficit hyperactivity disorder, there are many reasons why you might want to be highly sceptical. There is huge controversy about exactly who warrants this label and a widespread view that far too many people are being labelled.

The term 'attention deficit disorder' came to prominence not so long ago in 1980, when it was included in the psychiatrists' manual of mental disorders. And each time that manual has been updated since then, in 1987 and again in 1994, the definition of this disorder has changed, and expanded, to include more and more different behaviours, and catch more and more children in the net of illness.[6]

Definitions of disease are expanding all the time

The latest definition now includes 'symptoms' like: 'often fidgets with hands or feet', 'often easily distracted', and 'often has difficulty awaiting turn'. The obvious problem is that many of these are very normal behaviours for most energetic kids, so it is easy for parents, teachers or doctors to diagnose a disorder when there isn't one there. We are not suggesting here that ADHD does not exist or that some people may not benefit from treatment, but rather that it is an example of a disorder which, like many other disorders, has very rubbery and elastic boundaries. It's worth remembering too that some of the so-called experts who shout loudest about this disorder are taking money from the drug companies who make ADHD medications. Even some of the panels of experts who actually define this disorder have financial ties to the drug makers.

Expanding definitions of diseases have led to more and more people being diagnosed, and more and more people taking drugs. There are estimates now that in excess of 4 million Americans are using stimulant medications, including the well-known Ritalin and the newer drugs like Adderall. That includes 2.5 million children and 1.5 million adults. While these drugs have been shown to improve attention and focus, their long-term effects are unknown, and there are increasing concerns about the side effects of long-term use.[7]

In early 2006, advisers to the United States Food and Drug Administration met to discuss safety issues surrounding the use of ADHD drugs. These stimulant drugs increase heart rate and blood pressure, and there are growing concerns they could do damage as a result. The committee of high-level advisers discussed a small number of case reports of stroke, heart attack and sudden death in children and adults using these drugs. But despite the small number, there was enough concern for the committee to ask the powerful Food and Drug Administration to attach much stronger warnings to these drugs. In fact, the committee called for 'Black Box' warnings about these particular side effects, the strongest possible, to be attached. Importantly, they also felt that the drugs were being greatly overprescribed, and wanted to see their use more restricted.[8]

Another committee of advisers meeting a few months later did not recommend Black Box warnings, but did suggest adding more information to the label about possible heart-related and other side effects of these drugs.[9] Eventually the Food and Drug Administration did change the warnings—for some drugs they simply changed the label, for others they added a Black Box warning. For the popular drug Adderall, which is an amphetamine—a class of drugs sometimes known as 'speed'—Black Box warnings now include the following words: 'MISUSE OF AMPHETAMINE MAY CAUSE SUDDEN DEATH

AND SERIOUS CARDIOVASCULAR ADVERSE EVENTS.'[10] Other information on the Adderall label suggests that, even at usual doses, the drug may cause problems for kids who already have heart abnormalities.

With the emergence of a new disorder called 'adult ADHD', drug makers have identified a massive new market, and there has been a lot of hype about how many adults allegedly suffer this condition. According to the makers of Adderall, a pharmaceutical company called Shire, there are 8 million adults in the US who may need to be treated.[11] Shire sells almost US$1 billion worth of its drug annually already, making up half of the company's total sales.[12] The new warnings about Adderall and other ADHD drugs are very relevant for the many adults now being prescribed them as well as the children, whether it's in the United States, Australia or elsewhere. Research suggests that using amphetamines like Adderall can increase blood pressure to a level that in turn can increase your risk of heart disease and death.[13]

Already some doctors say they are spending a lot of time trying to reassure many patients they do not have the disorders that the patients have self-diagnosed in themselves or their kids. A recent survey of doctors in Australia suggested that many may spend up to one day a week trying to talk people out of thinking they have a disorder. One example that came up in the survey was ADHD—one-third of GPs suggested they often saw parents who had wrongly diagnosed ADHD in their kids.[14]

Often, in medicine, illness occurs as part of a spectrum from mild to severe. With conditions like ADHD, where there is potential for confusion between symptoms of the condition and ordinary life, it is worth making very sure there is something seriously wrong before you embrace a diagnosis and all the consequences that it can carry. Most people realise they have a choice about how to treat a disorder. Few realise they also have a choice about whether they accept that they have that disorder.

EXAMPLE 2
Osteoporosis

'Osteoporosis is a risk factor not a disease.' That was the simple title of a letter written to a British medical journal a few years ago by a London general practitioner.[15] In short, the

Being 'at risk' can be portrayed as a disease in itself

letter pointed out that if a person has osteoporosis, or low bone mineral density, that simply means they are at increased risk of fracture. It doesn't mean they are suffering a deadly disease. This is a view held by many people within the medical profession, but it is a view that you have probably never heard before. Why not? Those promoting the other view, that osteoporosis is a disease, have very loud voices and very deep pockets.[16]

If you can make everyone who is at risk of a disease fear that they actually have a disease, then urge them to see their doctors, get tested, and persuade them to take drugs for the rest of their lives, a lot of people will make a lot of money.

And that is pretty much what's happening with osteoporosis. Those benefiting include the doctors testing and treating that huge pool of osteoporosis 'patients', the companies that make the tests, and the corporations that sell the drugs. Fears about the 'silent killer' disease called osteoporosis have fuelled a giant global industry that is growing all the time.[17] The latest push is to make 'pre-osteoporosis' into a disease, a move which would instantly turn about half of all older women into patients.[18]

Before you decide to get your bones tested, and accept the label of a disease called osteoporosis, it is worth asking a few more questions. Questions like: 'Do I really need the test for this disease?'; 'Is this really a disease anyway, or just a risk factor?'; and 'Are there other things I can be doing to reduce my risks?'. The sorts of answers you can expect will depend a lot on your doctor and, in particular, how influenced he or she is by those pushing the drug solutions to preventing fractures.

In simple terms, osteoporosis is the loss of bone mass that tends to happen as we age, making fractures more likely. One of the problems here is with the actual definition. In 1994, a group of experts defining the 'disease' decided that 'normal' bone mass was the bone mass of a *young* woman.[19] What this meant was that a large number of older women were automatically defined as having a 'disease' called osteoporosis. This 'disease' is diagnosed using X-rays which measure a woman's bone mineral density at various parts of her body, like her neck or hip. If the bone density of the woman being X-rayed is a certain amount less than the bone density of a young woman, then the older woman is categorised as having osteoporosis. Clearly, this definition of osteoporosis instantly creates a huge potential market for osteoporosis drugs. Coincidentally, the meetings of those experts who defined the 'disease' back in 1994 were sponsored by the drug companies hoping to sell osteoporosis drugs to treat it.

The actual health problem here is a possible fracture, and how to prevent it. One of the big concerns is hip fractures, which can be devastating. Measuring someone's bone density is one way of trying to predict their risk of future fracture. For people who are at high risk of having a fracture, it may be a good thing to find out about that risk and do everything possible to reduce it—including taking drugs. But there are other factors that cause an increased risk of fracture, and getting too obsessed with bone density may distract us from those. Diet, exercise and alcohol-use all have an impact on a person's risk of falling or having a fracture, and there are obvious lifestyle changes that can reduce these risks. Relying only on bone density testing to predict future risk of fracture is by no means foolproof, and there is a growing discussion within the medical profession about the merits of relying less heavily on this measurement.[20]

Fractures are often caused by falls, and there are ways to try to prevent falls that have nothing to do with using osteoporosis drugs to build bone density. If we are interested in preventing fractures, then more time and effort would be spent trying to prevent falls among the elderly, but that wouldn't really make many people a lot of money. It would mean things like installing better lighting inside houses, removing slippery rugs, reducing prescription drug use and trying to get people doing more exercise. The obsession with bone density has come about because it is easily measured, and because there are drugs that increase it. For some, those drugs can reduce the risk of future fracture, though often only to a small extent.

As with many other disorders and diseases, we can be easily misled into thinking we have something wrong with us if we receive 'abnormal' test results. But with osteoporosis, the test results from a scan of your bones may not actually mean a lot in terms of your future risk of fracture. Because the results appear as hard numbers, both doctors and patients tend to give too much importance to them. As the London doctor wrote in his letter to the *British Medical Journal*: 'Bone density scanning is popular. It is popular with doctors and patients as it gives a number which they believe they understand.'[21]

There are similarities here between bone scans for osteoporosis and the PSA blood test for prostate cancer. As we learnt in the last chapter, the results of a PSA test may not actually mean a lot in terms of whether a man has prostate cancer or not. While doctors may try to make things sound very certain, there is usually a lot more uncertainty about what test results actually tell us. Pushing your doctor or other health professional to try to explain some of that uncertainty may stop you receiving a label you don't need, saving you from unnecessary anxiety as well as unnecessary tests and treatments.

As with ADHD, one of the key reasons to avoid being labelled with a disease called osteoporosis is that it can lead to lifelong drug use. For some people, particularly women at higher risks of fracture, there is evidence that some of the drugs can reduce the risk of having a fracture in a meaningful way. But it's important to remember that there is promising evidence that the risks of falling can most likely be reduced in other ways, such as through exercising, reducing drug and alcohol use, or changing diets, without having to ever consider yourself a patient or take long-term drugs.[22] For relatively healthy women at low risk, the label and the drugs that flow from it may do more harm than good. Several of the more popular drugs come with serious side effects, for example Fosamax can cause potentially severe problems in the oesophagus (between the mouth and stomach) and, in rare cases, problems affecting the jaw-bone.[23]

While osteoporosis is a multibillion dollar industry, there is a small but growing number of voices concerned that too many healthy women around the world are being told they are patients and put onto lifelong drug therapies which may do them more harm than good. Asking questions in a sceptical way about osteoporosis may be difficult, but could save you from unnecessary harm.

EXAMPLE 3
Female sexual dysfunction

The bigger the potential market of sick people, the more drugs you can sell. That's why drug companies are very interested in helping to relabel ordinary life as medical disease, a process that has been described as 'selling sickness' or 'disease-mongering'. The way drug companies have worked with doctors who are defining a new condition called female sexual dysfunction is a classic example of the corporate-sponsored creation of disease. Current

Sometimes new diseases are created

'definitions' suggest 43 per cent of women suffer from this condition, which is clearly an absurd claim.[24]

Believe it or not, there are now people working for drug companies who specialise in designing the way medical conditions like female sexual dysfunction are 'branded'. These are people with sophisticated skills in advertising, who help design the branding of drugs, but who actually specialise in branding the conditions too. Conditions like adult ADHD, erectile dysfunction, pre-menstrual dysphoric disorder, and social anxiety disorder have all been promoted to the public—particularly in the United States—as frightening new illnesses. Millions of ordinary people have seen full-page advertisements, watched commercials on TV and read stories in the paper about the latest epidemic. And much of that promotional activity has happened with help from those advertising gurus, experts in 'condition branding'. You don't have to take our word for it: one of those experts wrote an amazingly honest article about his work called 'The art of branding a condition', outlining how drug companies are involved in 'fostering the creation' of medical disorders.[25]

For more than a decade, a small group of scientists, doctors, psychologists and others have been meeting to refine and develop a definition of 'female sexual dysfunction.' Almost every meeting is heavily sponsored by the drug companies hoping to market a drug for this new condition. And companies are not just sponsoring the conferences and meetings: they are sending representatives along to them to build close relationships with the researchers defining this new illness. A few years ago, nineteen of these researchers sat down to write a definition, and eighteen of those people had financial ties to drug companies. At about the same time, a paper emerged suggesting 43 per cent of women suffer from this new condition. The researchers who produced that figure also had financial ties to the drug industry. That figure may be widely used in promotional material, but it has been discredited by other respected experts on female sexuality.

While the drug companies were busy sponsoring meetings about female sexual dysfunction, another group of researchers were developing a different view of female sexual difficulties. Driven by the feisty New York academic Dr Leonore Tiefer, this group has mounted a global campaign to expose the drug industry's involvement in defining this condition, publishing a book and other information offering a very different perspective on common sexual difficulties.[26] The researchers have pointed out that the 43 per cent figure is extremely unreliable. Rather than being an actual estimate of the percentage of women suffering a disease, it is simply an estimate of the number of healthy women who experience common sexual difficulties.

Despite such criticisms of the way in which this disease is being created, drug companies are racing to develop drugs to treat it as executives dream of enormous new markets. A recent business intelligence report prepared by a company called Datamonitor had this to say about the lucrative new disease: 'Datamonitor believes there is an opportunity to develop this market to parallel to that of the multibillion dollar male erectile dysfunction.'[27] As many readers will already know, erectile dysfunction became a huge market when the drug Viagra was launched in the late 1990s.

At this stage, only one drug to treat female sexual dysfunction has been approved, available in some European nations. Called Intrinsa, it is essentially testosterone for women. It is only a matter of time before more are approved, which will lead to an avalanche of promotional activity about this fearful 'disease'. For some women with a genuine medical problem, the label and the drugs—including Intrinsa—may be extremely valuable. For others they will be a useless, costly and dangerous distraction from the real sources of sexual dissatisfaction or difficulties. As one sex expert has written, the term 'dysfunction' is itself misleading, because the inhibition of sexual desire in many situations may be a perfectly healthy response. Promoting the existence of a widespread new disease may cause many women to think they have a dysfunction when they do not.

Conclusion
Do I really have that disorder?

Working out who is sick and who is healthy is not always as simple or straightforward as it might sound. When a child's face is covered with chickenpox, there is not a lot of doubt about what's wrong. But when a child fidgets in class, has trouble waiting their turn and talks excessively, do they have a medical disorder, family problems, or are they just an exuberant kid? Is it sufficient for a healthy fifty-something woman to keep exercising and eating well in order to reduce her risk of having a fall or fracture, or should she have her bones tested, accept the lifelong label of a disease called osteoporosis and go on potentially harmful drugs for the rest of her life? Is a thirty-something woman experiencing problems with her sex life suffering the symptoms of a dysfunction, or is she simply encountering the normal ups and downs of life? These are important questions worth asking.

Sometimes it is quite clear if someone is ill or has a disorder. In these cases, the sensible thing to do is to accept the diagnosis. But even then, it's important to ask questions like some of the others outlined in this book, such as: 'What are my options?' and 'How well does this treatment work?'. But the fact is there is sometimes far more uncertainty than we might assume surrounding whether or not we really do have a disorder or disease. In those cases it may be much better to reject an unhelpful medical label, and the medicines that usually go with it, and choose other ways to prevent illness and stay healthy.

More questions about disorders

Do I really have that disorder?

- Have the definitions of this disorder been expanding?
- Do I really need to be tested for that disease?
- Is this really a disease, or just a risk factor?
- If it is a risk factor, what is this likely to mean for my health, now or in the future?
- Are there other things I can do to reduce my risk?

Three

Do I really need to be screened?

'Screening' means testing healthy people to see if they have signs of disease. Some screening programs are valuable, but others are downright dangerous because too much testing can cause healthy people to be harmed unnecessarily. For this reason, it can be worthwhile asking questions about screening and hunting down answers before making any decisions. While breast cancer screening does seem worthwhile, its benefits have been oversold and are probably less than you might think. Screening for prostate cancer is widely promoted, but the scientific evidence suggests there is potential for it to do more harm than good. Meanwhile, there are concerns that some of those people promoting controversial screening tests for heart disease have serious financial conflicts of interest.

It seems like the most sensible thing in the world. Doctors, politicians, celebrities, even our friends and relations constantly urge us to get screened: to go and get tested for breast cancer, prostate cancer, heart disease and more. Newspapers and television shows are full of stories about the benefits of getting screened. Whatever the illness, surely it makes perfect sense to find it early, and treat it as aggressively as possible. Even the odd bit of inconvenience, like having your breasts squashed into a mammograph machine, is a small price to pay if that screening test is going to find a deadly cancer that can be successfully treated. After all, governments around the world pump millions of dollars into promoting regular screening tests. Surely anyone who questions a simple screening test would have to be a bit paranoid? In fact, there are very good reasons to ask questions about the pros and cons of screening programs.

One of the growing number of people who are asking such questions is Professor Simon Chapman, a leading public health researcher based at the University of Sydney. Professor Chapman has an international reputation for work on the harms of tobacco smoke, and he has sat on the board of the New South Wales Cancer Council for ten years. Like millions of middle-aged men all over the world, Simon Chapman is constantly being urged to 'be a man' and have a PSA test for prostate cancer—the test discussed in chapter 1. But unlike most men, he has had the opportunity to look behind a lot of the hype and read the scientific information about the benefits and harms for healthy men who do get screened for prostate cancer. 'I'm fifty-five years old and I haven't had a PSA screening test for prostate cancer,' he says. 'And for the moment, I have no intention of getting one.'[1]

One reason to ask questions is that some screening programs can actually inflict more harm than good, as may be the case with prostate cancer, the first example explored later in this chapter. Asking 'Do I really need to be screened?' may be well worth the trouble. Other screening programs have been shown to save lives, like screening for breast cancer. Yet it is important to know a little more about how many lives get saved, and to weigh up the benefits and harms of being screened. With breast cancer screening, you might be surprised to learn just how small those benefits are compared to the harms. Breast cancer screening is a great example of why we should ask, 'What are the actual benefits of getting screened?' And, finally, it is also good to know who is profiting from screening programs. If a screening program is funded by the government, you can generally assume it has some benefits. But when profit-driven clinics urge masses of healthy people to come in and get tested, it is worth being a little more sceptical, as we will see in the third example about testing your heart for calcium deposits. 'Who is profiting from this screening test?' is another key question to ask.

While screening has an important role to play in the health care system, many of us have an exaggerated sense of how helpful it can be. An international team of researchers published an article in the *British Medical Journal* in 2006, arguing that the public needed to be told a lot more about the pluses and minuses of undergoing a screening test.[2] The problem the team identified was that a lot of the information currently available is biased in favour of screening, and doesn't do a good job of informing people. The aim of much screening program information is to encourage people to be screened, rather than to ensure they fully understand the pros and cons. These researchers wrote that 'much current information overemphasises the benefits of screening, minimises the harms, and does not clarify to the reader that there is a choice to be made about whether screening is worthwhile for them'. Their article called for screening programs to be better evaluated, and for people to be told more about both the benefits and harms.

Urging healthy men to get screened for prostate cancer, for example, might seem like a sensible idea, but in fact many of the men who get tested may end up suffering more harm than good. That's because, with prostate cancer, for some men the treatments may be worse than the disease. Testing and treating prostate cancer is an extremely complex issue and it is very easy to be misled by people or organisations offering simplistic messages about the benefits of having a PSA test. While celebrities urging men to get tested might sound convincing, the hard science sends another message.[3]

Some screening programs do save lives, though the benefits may be less than you think

When groups of independent researchers go away and examine all the scientific information, they almost always reach the same conclusion. They find that, at this stage, recommending prostate cancer screening to men without any symptoms is the wrong thing to do. More evidence is needed before such a recommendation can be made. The more you learn about prostate cancer, the more Simon Chapman's view seems very reasonable.

Unlike prostate cancer screening, it is widely agreed that breast cancer screening extends lives.[4] Studies done around the world have found that women who undergo regular mammograms have lower risks of dying from breast cancer than women who don't get screened. But as we will learn later in this chapter, those risks are only lowered by a small amount. On the other side of the ledger, some women who are screened will have suspicious lumps investigated and be wrongly diagnosed as having cancer. At the end of the day, despite the complications and cost, many governments have been convinced that breast cancer screening is worthwhile. Despite its obvious benefits, you may like to weigh them up against the harms for yourself, and asking questions is one way to do that.

Using fear to sell products is one of the oldest tricks in the book, and the fear of heart attack is a particularly persuasive one. Many people will recall seeing advertisements urging healthy people to attend clinics testing their arteries for calcium deposits. These clinics and tests seem like a great idea, but rather than finding your fatty deposits, in our view another motivation for these clinics may well be building the bank deposits of the clinics' owners. In fact, these extensively advertised screening tests are highly controversial, and they have been heavily criticised by many

Some screening programs are heavily profit-driven

heart specialists. While looking for calcium in the arteries may help some people find out about their risks of heart attacks, the idea of urging every healthy person to undergo these tests may be extremely unhealthy.[5]

EXAMPLE 1
Prostate cancer screening

Screening healthy people may sometimes cause more harm than good

While celebrities and TV current affairs shows often urge healthy men to get tested for prostate cancer, many leading scientific bodies around the world do no such thing. Professor Simon Chapman recently decided to look more closely at this discrepancy and he was shocked by what he found. After doing a study of several years of newspaper stories and television news reports, he and his colleagues found that the overall message coming through the media supported the idea of prostate cancer screening. But when they looked at the recommendations of respected national and international medical organisations, they found there was an overwhelming view that there was not enough evidence to recommend in favour of screening. The media was tending to say one thing, while the scientific evidence was saying another.[6]

The International Union Against Cancer, the US Preventive Services Task Force, the UK National Screening Committee, the Australian Prostate Cancer Collaboration and the Australian Cancer Councils do *not* support screening the healthy population of men for prostate cancer, according to research done by Professor Chapman and his colleagues.[7] Similarly, a review of the studies of prostate cancer screening, published by the respected Cochrane Collaboration in 2006, concluded there was no good evidence available to help decide whether screening was worth it or not.[8] Unlike many other bodies, the American Cancer Society does recommend prostate cancer screening, reflecting a more aggressive approach that characterises the views of some medical groups in the United States.[9]

Contrasting the promotion of screening that comes from television and newspaper reports with the cautious approach of the scientific bodies, the University of Sydney researcher was outraged. 'This coverage was grossly misleading by omission,' says Simon Chapman. 'Men are not being given enough information to help balance the enthusiastic endorsements they are hearing.'[10]

Because more and more men are being tested, more and more men are being diagnosed with prostate cancer. In fact, it is now the most commonly diagnosed cancer in men in Australia, leading people to think it's the biggest killer—which it is not.[11] Prostate cancer is the sixth leading cause of death amongst men, says Simon Chapman, a fair way behind heart attacks and strokes. Prostate cancer also tends to kill men very late in life, so when you compare all the diseases in terms of actual number of years of life lost, prostate cancer comes in at ninth place. The concern about the increasing rates of diagnosis is that much of it may be unnecessary.

It is clear that prostate cancer can kill, with around 3000 Australian men dying of the disease every year, which is more than the number of women who die from breast cancer.[12] It is also clear that for some men the treatments will prevent the terrible symptoms of the illness. For example, a major Scandinavian study published in the *New England Journal of Medicine* compared surgery with 'watchful waiting'—meaning not undertaking surgery immediately—for men with early prostate cancer. That study found that over six years, fewer men died of prostate cancer specifically in the group given surgery (though overall survival rates were similar for the two groups).[13]

The problem is that there is much uncertainty about who should be treated, and whether for some people the treatment may do more harm than good. Because it is often slow-growing, many men have cancer in their prostates that will never actually harm them, and they will die of something else first. As a consequence, some men are having cancers removed that may never have threatened their lives. The nature of this cancer is that the more we look for it in healthy men, the more we are likely to find it. This problem is sometimes called overdiagnosis, and it is of great concern. Some researchers have suggested that perhaps one-half of the cases of cancer picked up through PSA testing would not have otherwise been picked up in the man's lifetime.[14]

The biggest concern about overdiagnosis is that some men will be unnecessarily subjected to the treatments for prostate cancer, which can carry major complications. There is a lot of debate about exactly how common these complications are. Reliable research suggests, however, that for men undergoing radical surgery, around 15 per cent or more of them may end up incontinent and between 20 and 80 per cent of them may end up with erection problems, not to mention the normal risks associated with major surgery including infections and even, in very rare circumstances, death.[15] If the treatment is going to extend life in a meaningful way, these complications may well be worth it. If the treatment was not needed in the first place, they are entirely unnecessary. The trouble is, it's hard to know what's needed and what's not, because it isn't always easy to predict whether a man's cancer is going to go on to kill him or not.

Healthy men who undertake a PSA test for prostate cancer are taking a risk that they may ultimately be treated for a cancer that would never have hurt them. But on the other hand, healthy men, without symptoms, who have decided not to have a PSA test—men like Simon Chapman—are also taking a risk, as he explains: 'For my own case, I'm willing to let sleeping dogs lie. I may have an aggressive cancer inside of me, but I may not. My reading of the scientific information is that it's probably best if I don't have the PSA test. The gamble that I'm taking, is that one day I might be diagnosed with an aggressive cancer, which if I had been tested earlier may have been picked up—but we'll never actually know that.'[16] The decision is complicated and, given how high the stakes are, it's a decision well worth considering carefully, and asking questions about. Decision aids like those discussed in chapter 4, 'What are my options?', may well help.

EXAMPLE 2
Breast cancer screening

Weighing up benefits and harms Unlike prostate cancer, there is strong evidence suggesting that if the healthy population of older women is tested for breast cancer, potentially deadly cancers will be found and some peoples' lives will be extended as a result. Backed by this evidence, breast screening programs—also known as mammography—continue to win widespread support around the world and they are often heavily funded and promoted by governments. In Australia, as part of a publicly funded program, women aged fifty to sixty-nine are urged to have breast X-rays every two years, and in the United States there is a big push from some quarters for women to be screened from age forty.

Like almost everything in medicine, there are downsides to breast cancer screening, so weighing up benefits and harms may be a valuable thing to do. In this case that means asking: 'What are the actual benefits of screening?' and 'What are the harms of getting screened?' The short answer, according to the evidence we are about to explore, is that only a relatively small number of the many women who get screened will benefit directly by having their deadly cancers removed, and a slightly higher number of women will be harmed by undergoing aggressive treatment which they would never have needed.

The longer answer, for those who have a stomach for numbers, goes like this. A recent review of all the studies suggests that women over fifty who are regularly screened for ten years end up reducing their risk of dying from breast cancer, in relative terms, by about 15 to 20 per cent, compared to women who don't get screened.[17] That figure does sound impressive, but it is a figure expressing benefits in *relative* terms. As we will discuss later in chapter 5, 'How well does that treatment work?', when you express statistics in *relative* terms, they tend to sound more impressive than they really are. If you express them in *absolute* terms, the numbers often sound a little less convincing.

According to this high-quality systematic review, screening reduces an individual woman's chances of dying from breast cancer, in *absolute* terms, by only around 0.05 per cent, or five in ten thousand.[18] Put another way, for every 2000 women invited to be screened over a ten-year period, one woman will have her deadly cancer discovered and successfully treated, and her life will be extended as a result. Unfortunately no one can say which woman will be the lucky one, or by how much her life will be extended. It could be days, it could be years. A separate study from Scandinavia, which was recently analysed by researchers from Britain, is more optimistic about the benefits of screening.[19] It suggests that for every 250 women screened, one life will be extended. Such differing estimates of the benefits of screening may seem strange but are actually commonplace in medicine, where there is often great uncertainty about how well things work.

On the harms side of the equation, as with prostate cancer screening, breast cancer screening will find some early cancers that would never have proved deadly, and did not need to be treated in the first place. In other words, a number of women will be overdiagnosed and treated unnecessarily. Working out exactly how many women will be treated unnecessarily is not easy, and there are varying estimates, depending on which study you look at. The systematic review of all studies mentioned above suggests that for every 2000 women invited to be screened over a ten-year period, ten healthy women will be overdiagnosed and treated for breast cancer unnecessarily. That means that for every 2000 women screened for ten years, one will have their life extended and ten will be treated unnecessarily. The authors of this systematic review, who happen to be known worldwide for both their scepticism and their scientific rigour, conclude: 'It is not clear whether screening does more harm than good. Women invited to screening should be fully informed of both benefits and harms.'[20]

The analysis of the Scandinavian study, which is more optimistic about benefits, is also very clear about the potential harms. It suggests that for every 250 women screened, one will have her life extended, and two women will be treated unnecessarily.[21] The authors of this more optimistic analysis suggest that the unnecessary treatment suffered by some women is 'part of the price' of saving the lives of other women. A surgeon commenting on the pros and cons of breast cancer screening in the *British Medical Journal* puts it this way: 'Although breast screening by mammography is far from perfect, it is worthwhile.'[22]

As is obvious from the differing views, benefits and harms are not always clear-cut and can be interpreted differently by different experts, so it is worthwhile asking questions. Whichever numbers are ultimately proved to be accurate, it seems that for breast screening, there are both positives and negatives to be weighed up.

For women under fifty it's a different story again, and the potential benefits of screening are smaller and even less clear. In Australia, the government-backed screening program is targeted at women aged between fifty and sixty-nine, but women under fifty are able to be tested if they want to. In the United States there is a significant push from some groups to screen women from forty years of age. Researchers at the University of Sydney have looked at all the evidence about the benefits and harms of breast screening for women between forty and fifty and have written a 'decision aid' for people, which is available for free on the Internet. As the researchers write, 'A decision aid is intended to provide you with unbiased information so that you can make a decision after considering the evidence.'[23] (Decision aids are further discussed in chapter 4, 'What are my options?'.)

In brief, the decision aid compares what will happen to women who start getting screened at age forty with those who don't get screened during their forties. Of 2000 women who begin screening at forty, roughly four will ultimately die from breast cancer. Of those who don't get screened, roughly five will die from breast cancer. That's means there is a potential benefit of preventing death and extending life. But what else will happen to those women being screened during their forties? Of the 2000 women who are screened, roughly 480 of them will have extra tests because their mammogram was 'abnormal'. While these tests will ultimately show they do not have cancer, 'some women will worry long after they have had them,' according to the researchers. These figures may seem a little confusing, so consider taking a look at the decision aid if you are interested in learning more, as it uses easy-to-understand diagrams. Discussing this with a friend or loved one might also help.[24]

The authors of this decision aid do not make a recommendation to women in their forties, other than saying this:

> Many people think mammograms to detect breast cancer early are always a good thing. But there are reasons why you might choose not to start screening mammography if you are younger than 50 . . . Remember there is no right or wrong answer about whether to start having screening. It is your decision to make.[25]

Given the massive amount of publicity supporting breast cancer screening, many women will understandably undergo mammography without feeling the need to ask too many questions. But like all medical interventions, breast screening comes with downsides. Getting in the habit of asking questions can't be a bad thing.

EXAMPLE 3
Heart screening for calcium

The headline at the top of the press release was dramatic: 'New approach could prevent 90 000 sudden cardiac deaths and save $21 billion annually.'[26] A report by an international task force of heart experts was advocating a revolutionary new plan to screen all healthy men from age forty-five and all women from age fifty-five to find out who was at risk of a heart attack. One of the tests promoted by the task force was a CT scan that is used to look inside arteries for calcium, one of the components of the plaque that builds up and raise the risk of heart attack. Many clinics offer these sorts of tests and have been advertising them widely for several years, urging healthy people to check out their risk of heart attack. It seems like such a sensible idea. What on earth could be wrong with this radical new plan to screen everyone and dramatically reduce heart attacks?

Watch out for vested interests

If we ask 'Who's profiting from this screening test?', the answer can be very helpful. If millions more people are discovered to be at risk of heart disease, then one group to benefit will be the pharmaceutical companies that sell heart drugs. As it turns out, a line near the bottom of the press release, mentioned above, reveals that the report which was calling for mass heart screening of healthy people was funded by Pfizer, the biggest drug company in the world and maker of the heart medicine Lipitor, one of the most heavily marketed and commercially successful drugs of all time. But it was not just the drug company sponsorship which suggests the need for scepticism about the report and its radical new plan: the report has also been criticised for not accurately reflecting the scientific evidence about the value of heart screening. A news story about the report in the *British Medical*

Journal carried highly critical comments, suggesting its recommendations to screen the entire older population were not based on strong evidence.[27]

The group behind the drug company-funded report is called Screening for Heart Attack Prevention and Education, or SHAPE. According to its website, one of SHAPE's three 'partner' groups is an organisation called the Boomer Coalition, but there is no mention of where this organisation gets its money.[28] On the surface, the Boomer Coalition looks like a grassroots group of baby boomers concerned about fighting heart disease. In fact, the Boomer Coalition began life a few years ago as a public relations creation—initially funded by Pfizer to the tune of US$10 million.[29]

Along with the drug companies selling heart drugs, doctors running the heart clinics offering scans would also benefit enormously if every healthy middle-aged person started getting regular CT scans that check their arteries for calcium. So while it is clear those promoting these tests will benefit, it is not at all clear how much those getting tested will benefit. When independent groups look at the scientific evidence they have come to very different conclusions than those offered in the drug company–sponsored report.

For example, the United States Preventive Services Task Force, which is publicly funded, wrote a report on heart screening in 2004, and recommended against testing healthy people at low risk of heart attack and stroke.[30] According to the report, the problem with a mass screening program is that many healthy people will receive test results indicating they may have a problem when in fact they do not. And that means many people will undergo costly and invasive tests they didn't need. In other words, there will be a lot of 'false positive' test results.

The US Preventive Services Task Force found that these false positive test results are 'likely to cause harm, including unnecessary invasive procedures, over-treatment, and labelling' and they concluded that in adults at low risk, 'the potential harms of routine screening . . . exceed the potential benefits'. For adults at higher risk, the report concluded that there was not enough evidence to make a recommendation and therefore 'could not determine the balance between benefits and harms of screening'. The point is not that these CT tests for calcium are of no value: in fact they may have a useful role in helping diagnose and treat heart disease in some people at increased risk. The point is that the evidence does not yet support recommending them to every healthy older person. This approach may well do more harm than good.[31]

Apart from leading to further tests or treatments that may be unnecessary, the CT scans themselves can cause direct harm, most importantly raising the risk of cancer, as we discussed in chapter 1. A study published in the *Journal of the American Medical Association* in 2007 warned that women and young people in particular need to be aware of the increased cancer risk associated with undergoing CT scans, which are frequently being used to check people's arteries for the presence of calcium.[32] There is already concern in Australia about the overuse of CT scans of the chest. In all the debate about scans, it's important to remember that very established methods exist to work out a person's risk of heart attack and how to effectively lower it—like changing diet or doing more exercise.

Conclusion

Do I really need to be screened?

Asking questions about complex matters like screening programs may seem daunting. But, as we have learnt, a lot of what you read, see and hear overemphasises the benefits of screening and plays down the harms. With prostate cancer screening and heart screening, there are many self-interested advocates among the medical profession, the test manufacturers and the drug makers who urge everyone to get regularly tested. It is only when more independent groups and individuals like Professor Simon Chapman take a long, hard look at the evidence that they find these screening programs may do more harm than good.

Unlike other medical interventions, screening tests are given to healthy people: people who have no symptoms, are not yet sick, and may not get sick for a long time. When someone is ill they are more prepared to risk the possible complications of tests or treatments, particularly if there is good evidence that their treatment might help fix their illness. But for healthy people there is no disease that needs fixing, so the risks of the screening tests really need to be very, very low and the benefits must outweigh their harms in a meaningful way. For some screening procedures—like breast cancer screening—that seems to be case, though there is still a lively debate about this issue. For some other screening programs, we are a long way from having convincing evidence that benefits outweigh harms.

More questions about screening

Do I really need to be screened?

- What are the harms of being screened?
- What are the benefits of being screened?
- What are the sorts of tests and treatments that might follow if the initial screening test is positive?
- What are the benefits and harms of those subsequent tests and treatments?
- What are the chances that the screening test will find a disease that would never have actually caused me any harm?
- Who is profiting from this screening test?

QUESTIONS ABOUT YOUR TREATMENT

Four

What are my options?

You cannot always rely on doctors or other health professionals to tell you about the full range of options available for treating or managing illnesses and other health problems. One option in particular is often overlooked—the fact that many common conditions may not require treatment at all. Similarly, 'watchful waiting'—delaying a decision about whether to start treatment—is often not mentioned as an option. Written materials called 'decision aids' can help you to weigh up the pros and cons of all your options. Using a decision aid may lead you to make quite different choices about your care than you otherwise might.

The way patients interact with doctors and other health professionals is undergoing a profound revolution. In the past, many people went to doctors expecting to be told what tests or treatments to have. These days, more and more people are expecting to have a say in the decisions that affect their health. And many researchers and health professionals support such a shift and have been working to develop tools to help patients play a greater role in making these decisions.

But not all health professionals have caught up with this revolution, which has been called the move towards 'patient-informed decision making'. Lacking the skills or attitudes to help patients play a greater role in their health care decisions, some are still stuck in old-fashioned ways. Nor do all patients want to take on the extra thought and effort involved; some people are quite happy to be told what to do—whether to have an operation or to take a particular medicine, for example. And sometimes patients and their families may not be able to be involved in making decisions for practical reasons, such as in emergencies.

If you do want to have a greater say in your health care, you need to understand what your options are and how to weigh them up. Many people confronting an illness assume there must be 'one right way' of treating or managing it. Sometimes, that is the case. But often there is much uncertainty about what is the best approach out of a number of available options, all with different pros and cons needing to be weighed up. And you can't always rely on health professionals to tell you about all the options and their pros and cons. The first example, on back pain, later in this chapter demonstrates that the options offered may vary according to the type of health professional you see: not surprisingly, you may be more likely to end up having surgery if you consult a surgeon rather than a physiotherapist. The options on offer might also vary according to where you live; people living in country areas or poorer suburbs might not have access to the same range of treatments available elsewhere.

It can be a mistake to assume that health professionals will always suggest the best and most effective treatment for your problem. Like anyone else, health professionals become used to

Be proactive in seeking out your options

doing things the way they have always done them, and so might still be recommending treatments that are not supported by the latest evidence. Or they may be so overwhelmed with information that they can't keep up with the most recent evidence about the best treatments. They may even be watching the clock, conscious of the many other patients in their waiting room and unable to take the time needed to make sure you understand all the options available to you.

There are also many vested interests—like drug companies and surgical device manufacturers—encouraging health professionals to use a particular test or treatment for commercial reasons (read more about this in chapter 9, 'Who else is profiting here?'). On the other side of the coin, governments, private health insurers and other funding bodies may not cover all of the treatments that might be effective for your condition.

So you need to be proactive in seeking out information about your options. You also need to be aware that doing nothing is one important but often overlooked option for some common health complaints. Many conditions will resolve of their own accord without the need for any treatment, as is illustrated in the back pain example. A related option is watchful waiting, knowing that you may choose to be treated at a later stage if you don't get better. One of the benefits of this approach, as illustrated in the second example's examination of antibiotic use in children, is that you may be able to avoid the cost and inconvenience associated with some treatments, not to mention the risk of side effects.

One of the reasons that patients may not be given the option of no treatment or watchful waiting is the natural human tendency to want to act when faced with a problem. Health professionals often find it difficult to resist the temptation to act; sometimes they assume patients expect to be given a treatment and might feel deprived if simply told to do nothing. This is particularly likely when parents are anxious about their children. And you might find that well-meaning family members or friends also push you to 'do something', perhaps not appreciating that a conscious decision not to have any treatment is often a valid option. Sometimes, someone needs to shout out: 'Don't just do something, stand there!'

Considering your options means more than simply identifying the choices that are available. You also need to understand the potential benefits and harms of each option, and how important these are to you in your current situation. Different people may weigh up these factors quite differently. What counts is what is important to you. It can be very confusing for any one person to get a grip on all the options in front of them, and that's why information tools known as decision aids are becoming increasingly common.

Good decision aids spell out all the options available to patients and explain the potential benefits and harms of each option in language that is easy to understand. They then allow you to rate the options according to your own situation and preferences, as demonstrated in the third example on breast cancer. But decision aids cannot always tell you everything you would like to know, partly because we don't have answers for all the questions that arise in health care. Patients and health professionals often have to make decisions in the face of considerable uncertainty. Even when there is good evidence about what benefit or harm a treatment might impart, there still remains uncertainty about how these may play out for any individual. Often the best that a decision aid can tell you is how likely it is that a particular benefit or side effect will occur. This is not a guarantee of how you personally will be affected.

While guarantees are rare in health care, taking the time and effort to explore the full range of available options may result in you receiving the health care that is best suited to your needs and situation. You may also feel more satisfied about your care if you've been actively involved in making the decisions.

EXAMPLE 1
Back pain

Most people suffer from back pain at least once in their lives, and many will experience it multiple times. The pain can become excruciating, making everyday tasks extremely challenging. Being in the midst of a bad bout of back pain can be frightening, and it can feel difficult to imagine that life will ever again return to normal.

Checking out your options might save you from harmful tests and treatments

When you are in pain and anxious, it can also be tempting to try any sort of help that is on offer, whether it is recommended by a health professional or friend. Even if they are well-meaning, their advice could make things worse rather than better. Back pain provides a compelling example of why it is important to ask plenty of questions about your options, and find out about their potential harms and benefits.

It is important to understand what doctors call the 'natural history' of your condition. This means understanding what you can expect to happen if you do nothing. When it comes to back pain, the reality is that most people will make a full recovery from an acute episode, with most pain and related disability resolving within a couple of weeks. Only about five per cent of people—or about one in every twenty—who suffer an acute episode will go on to have long-term pain and disability.[1] Understanding this may influence what treatments you are prepared to consider: with such a good chance of recovery anyway, many people may be less willing to have treatments which involve risk or expense.

On a similar note, about 90 per cent of people with back pain have no identifiable cause for their problem.[2] This suggests that many people undergo unnecessary tests for back pain; for most people, there will be no point having a test because it will not be able to find any cause. As discussed in Question 1, 'Do I really need that test?', there are many reasons to avoid having unnecessary tests, including the risk of 'false positive' results. In other words, MRI scans will often give a 'positive' result, even when the person having the scan doesn't have back pain. It's also sensible to avoid unnecessary tests like CT scans, which use high doses of radiation.

Whether your back pain is a one-off acute episode or a long-term chronic problem, understanding your condition and all the available treatment options is vital for maximising your chances of recovery. This is particularly important as approaches to managing back pain vary enormously. Despite there often being no obvious cause to 'fix', a wide range of professionals have become involved in treating back pain, including surgeons, occupational physicians, physiotherapists, chiropractors, osteopaths and acupuncturists, to name just a few. This has led to a proliferation of different treatment approaches, some of which are unlikely to help and may even do harm.

Many people have been advised, for example, to take long periods off work and to rest, although this approach can actually slow recovery by weakening the muscles that support the spine and making you stiffer and less fit. It can also reinforce peoples' perceptions of themselves as disabled rather than encouraging them to remain active, which helps with recovery. Many people have also undergone surgery unnecessarily, involving a significant risk of complications, which may be as serious as paralysis of the legs. Indeed, one Australian study suggests that back operations are a major cause of serious complications in private hospitals.[3] This is particularly worrying given concerns that many of these operations may be unnecessary and sometimes represent 'overservicing'.

Because so many different types of professionals have been involved in managing back pain, it has taken many years to work out what approaches are most likely to help. Patients' best interests have sometimes been lost in the arguments between various professional groups over who knows best. Patients have only really started to benefit when all of the professionals with an interest in back pain have started to work together. This sort of cooperative approach—which happens too rarely in the health sector—has led to the development of a number of evidence-based guidelines for both acute and chronic back pain. These are more reliable than recommendations driven by just one professional group as guidelines prepared by surgeons, for example, may be more likely to recommend surgery as an option. It's a reminder of the importance of asking: 'Are there any clinical practice guidelines or reviews by reputable bodies that might help explain my options?'

In a nutshell, these evidence-based guidelines recommend that people with acute back pain—or pain which has just started—should be reassured about their good chances of recovery, advised to stay active, and prescribed medication or behavioural treatment (psychological therapies aimed at helping people change how they perceive and respond to their problems) for pain relief, if necessary. They may also consider having spinal manipulation for pain relief and should not be advised to have bed rest or to do special exercises for their backs.

Guidelines for chronic back pain—or pain which lasts over a long period—strongly recommend exercise and intensive multidisciplinary pain treatment programs. They say there is some evidence to support the effectiveness of various medications, spinal manipulation and psychological therapies to change the way people think about and respond to their back pain. And the guidelines highlight a lack of reliable studies to evaluate the effects of many commonly used interventions, including surgery and steroid injections.

The point of mentioning all these options is not to imply that you should try one over another. The aim is to highlight that many treatment options are often available, some of which are backed up by good research evidence and some of which are not. Your GP or other health professional may not have the time, inclination or ability to explain the pros and cons of all the available options; you may need to do some research yourself. Luckily the Internet provides easy access to reliable sources of information about back pain management (see box). The example of back pain management illustrates the importance of asking your doctor: 'What happens if I do nothing?' and 'What is the natural history of this condition for someone like me?'

For more information about back pain:

- *BMJ* Clinical Evidence: <www.clinicalevidence.org>
- Cochrane Back Review Group: <www.cochrane.iwh.on.ca>
- European Commission Guidelines: <www.backpaineurope.org>

EXAMPLE 2
Children's infections

Parents need to understand watchful waiting

No one likes to see a child suffering with an illness. The natural reaction for many people, whether they are parents or the family doctor, is to want to do something to relieve the pain and suffering. This natural instinct is reinforced by companies that market medicines for children, using strategies which play heavily on parental fears.

So it is not surprising that most children end up being prescribed antibiotics at some stage, often for such common complaints as colds, middle ear infections, sore throats, runny noses and conjunctivitis. There is growing concern, however, about this widespread use of antibiotics, especially for problems that will often resolve of their own accord without any treatment. The concerns are twofold. First of all, antibiotics, like any medicine, involve a risk of side effects. Usually these are minor and don't last long, like nausea, vomiting or diarrhoea, but occasionally they can be more serious. Many children may be suffering side effects but not deriving any significant benefit from the drugs. The second important concern about the widespread use of antibiotics for minor complaints is that it is contributing to the spread of germs that are resistant to antibiotic treatment. This means that it is becoming increasingly difficult to treat patients with more serious and potentially even life-threatening conditions because the drugs are losing their power to fight bacteria.

In recent times, these concerns have driven a major rethink of the use of antibiotics to treat minor childhood complaints. Several important studies called 'randomised controlled trials' have compared the potential benefits and harms of three different approaches to treating childhood infections. (See chapter 8, 'What is the evidence?', to learn more about these studies.) The approaches include: giving antibiotics, giving no treatment at all, and giving treatment at a later stage if symptoms have not improved. The results illustrate why it is important that parents and doctors consider their options before rushing to dose kids with antibiotics.

These studies show that most children will recover from conditions such as uncomplicated middle ear infection, conjunctivitis, colds and runny noses whether they have antibiotics or not. While antibiotics may speed up their recovery slightly, this benefit needs to be weighed up against the risk of side effects. For example, children are as likely to suffer side effects from taking antibiotics for a pussy runny nose or middle ear infection as they are likely to be helped by them.[4]

Traditionally, the justification for using antibiotics to treat common conditions was because of the risk of very rare but serious complications, such as rheumatic fever. However, these complications are so rare that a growing number of researchers and doctors question the wisdom of exposing almost all children to the risks of side effects of antibiotics in order to prevent these very rare problems. They believe it makes much more sense to target the use of antibiotics towards those children who are at greatest risk of serious complications from the infection and employ watchful waiting for the others. In many countries, for example, health authorities now recommend that children with acute middle ear infection should not generally be prescribed antibiotics immediately, and that a 'wait and see' policy be adopted.[5]

But old habits die hard, and not all doctors are convinced of the merits of this sort of approach. Many continue to automatically dispense antibiotics for the common complaints of childhood, an approach which has been branded as 'excessive interference by the medical profession'.[6] An added obstruction is that many parents do not appreciate that conditions like conjunctivitis will generally get better of their own accord.

The message here is not that children should never have antibiotics for these conditions but that it should be a carefully considered decision. After weighing up the pros and cons of all these options, you might decide to use the antibiotics. Many people do—even in the clinical trials mentioned above, many parents asked for antibiotics for their children, even though they were not offered by the treating doctor. You may consider, for example, that if antibiotics can cut the duration of your child's illness by even half a day, this is worth it, especially if it means they can attend day care.

But if antibiotics are suggested for your child, it is at least worth asking the questions: 'What happens if I do nothing?' and 'Is watchful waiting an option?' And these are also questions well worth asking when it comes to your own health care generally.

EXAMPLE 3
Breast cancer

In the early 1980s, surgeons were confronted by two important studies challenging what was then accepted as the best way of treating women who had been diagnosed with an early breast cancer. At that time,

Getting informed using 'decision-aids' may change your health care

most women with early breast cancer were told that radical mastectomy—a major operation to remove the entire breast and surrounding tissue—was their only treatment option. It resulted in significant scarring, and could also cause long-term complications.

The studies challenging the accepted wisdom created a sensation because they suggested that women with breast cancer could avoid having such major surgery and be just as successfully treated by less invasive surgery, combined with radiotherapy. Since those landmark studies were published, a number of other good trials have confirmed these results. They also suggest that women treated with the less invasive breast-conserving surgery plus radiation are more likely to feel satisfied with their treatment and to report a better quality of life.

But, as we've already discussed, old habits die hard amongst the medical profession. Many women continued to have the more invasive radical surgery. Sometimes this was because they'd made an informed choice—they decided they would prefer to have major surgery than to undergo radiotherapy.

But often it was because they did not realise they had more than one option. Or, if they did realise this, they did not fully understand the implications of each option.

Concerns that women were not being fully informed about their options led to the development of decision aids to help them and their doctors better negotiate the breast cancer treatment maze. There was also the recognition that people are upset and fearful when receiving a traumatic diagnosis like cancer and may not fully comprehend the options they are being given, so decision aids can help by providing a more structured and systematic approach to delivering information. They also encourage patients to reflect upon how the pros and cons of their different options weigh up for them personally. Decision aids don't yet exist for all diseases and conditions, but there are a growing number available.

To find decision aids:

- **Ottawa Health Research Institute Patient Decision Aids Research Group: <decisionaid.ohri.ca/decaids.html>**
- **Dartmouth-Hitchcock Medical Center: <www.dhmc.org>**
- **Sydney Health Decision Group: <www.health.usyd.edu. au/shdg>**

The potential benefits of decision aids were highlighted in a Canadian study in which surgeons were randomly allocated to two different groups. Each group used a different way of giving information to women newly diagnosed with early breast cancer: either using decision aids or following their normal procedures for delivering information. The study found that if their surgeon used a decision aid to communicate with their patients, the women were more likely to choose the less invasive breast-conserving surgery plus radiation, rather than radical surgery. They were also more likely to be well-informed about their options, to feel less uncertainty, to feel that they had been offered a clear choice and to be more satisfied with their decision making.[7]

The researchers in the Canadian study concluded that decision aids can improve doctor–patient communication and decision making. Many other studies have also suggested that patients who are well-informed by a decision aid sometimes make quite different decisions from those who are not so well-informed.[8]

So, if you are facing a decision about your health care, it is worth asking the question: 'Are there any decision aids which spell out the pros and cons of the various options?' It's also worth asking who has developed the decision aid. It may not be as reliable if funded by a pharmaceutical company or any other group with a vested interest in pushing a particular treatment. If you can't find any helpful, independent decision aids, look for clinical practice guidelines produced by independent groups. (See chapter 8, 'What is the evidence?', for more information about such guidelines.)

Conclusion

What are my options?

Too often, patients are not fully informed about all of the options that might be available to them. Even if they are told about the options that are available, they may not be given helpful information about the pros and cons of each option and how these may affect them personally, taking into account their individual situation. Patients are particularly unlikely to be told if having no treatment or watchful waiting are realistic options for their situation.

Sometimes this is because there is only one realistic option available. Sometimes there is not the time or opportunity for patients to be involved in making decisions about their health care. But there is growing evidence that people might make quite different decisions about what tests or treatments to have if they are fully informed about the pros and cons of all their options.

Investigating your options fully could save you from having unnecessary, costly or even harmful tests and treatments. It may also lead to you having treatments that are more effective and more suited to your needs and personal preferences. You can't assume you will always be told of all the available options. It's up to you to ask about them.

More questions about your options

What are my options?

- What are the pros and cons of not having treatment?
- What happens if I do nothing?
- What is the natural history of this condition for someone like me?
- Is watchful waiting an option?
- Are there any decision aids that spell out the pros and cons of the various options?
- Are there any clinical practice guidelines or reviews by reputable bodies that might help explain my options?

Five

How well does that treatment work?

Every day, many people around the world undergo treatments that are unlikely to be helpful. These treatments might be medicines, complementary therapies, surgical operations or other procedures. Just because treatments are available and recommended does not mean they will help. The benefits of many widely used treatments are often questionable and, even if they do work, are frequently overpromoted. Many treatments may be more than just a waste of your money and time—they may be more likely to do harm than good. To make sure you have treatments that work means being prepared to ask the question—and sometimes repeatedly: 'How well does that treatment work?'

Many treatments are not as effective as you might expect. If they have not been carefully evaluated there is often great uncertainty about how helpful they might be, or even whether they are helpful at all. And in cases where studies *have* suggested that a treatment is beneficial, the results may not be reliable, as many evaluations of treatments are of poor quality.

There are several reasons why everyone—whether patient or doctor—tends to have an overly optimistic view of treatments. For a start, much of the research into treatments is funded by pharmaceutical companies or others with a vested interest in promoting a particular product. It has been well-documented that studies funded by vested interests are more likely to be biased, overplaying the benefits of treatments and underplaying the harms.[1] As well, studies concluding that a treatment works are more likely to be submitted and accepted for publication than studies showing that a treatment is unlikely to have any benefit, or is actually harmful. The

Benefits of treatments can be exaggerated

news media, in turn, is more likely to report on studies showing benefit from a treatment. The headline 'New cancer drug makes no difference' is not considered as newsworthy as 'New cancer drug saves lives'. It's no wonder we so often end up with an overly optimistic picture.

Even when a treatment has been proven to make a positive difference, this doesn't mean it will benefit everyone who has it. Hardly any treatments have 100 per cent success rates. So you need to find out what is the chance or probability that any treatment might make a difference to you. It's not enough to ask: 'Does that treatment work?' You need to ask: 'How well does that treatment work?'

Often the impact of treatments is expressed in a way that makes it seem much more dramatic than it really is. It sounds pretty impressive if you hear that a new drug has produced a 20 per cent increase in cure rates. But what that actually means may not be so impressive when you look more closely. It may mean, for example, that if a hundred people take the drug for several years, twelve will be cured, compared with ten being cured if the drug wasn't taken. That's a 20 per cent increase in *relative* terms, but a 2 per cent increase in *absolute* terms. And you may also need to balance the fact that if a hundred people take the drug for several years, many will suffer serious side effects in order for those extra two people to be cured. So you can't afford to take claims about the benefits of treatments on face value; you need to ask questions to find out exactly what is known about how well a treatment works. You could ask, for example: 'How many people need to take a treatment, in order for one person to benefit?' In the hypothetical drug example above, a hundred people may have to be treated for two people to benefit. Or you could ask: 'How likely is it that the treatment will help me?'

It is not only the pharmaceutical industry that has done such a good job of overselling the benefits of its products. The complementary health sector is also skilled at overplaying its hand. For instance, the vitamins known as antioxidants have been widely promoted for their supposed benefits in warding off a range of problems, from heart disease to cancer. But, as revealed in the first example in this chapter, their benefits have been way oversold. Antioxidants are not only ineffective in preventing many of these diseases, but some may be downright harmful.

If you are sick, you cannot assume that you will be told about or offered the treatment most likely to be of help. The health care industry is often set up in a way that favours the use of treatments such as medicines over other remedies which may be just as helpful or even more so. Many forces combine to promote pill-pushing as the solution for health problems when other approaches—such as psychological therapies or lifestyle changes—might be better. This has certainly been the case with dementia treatments, where much funding and effort has gone into developing and promoting medicines that have only a modest impact on patients' well-being, as illustrated in the second example in this chapter. It's a reminder of the importance of asking: 'Are there any other treatment options that don't involve taking pills?'

Just because a doctor prescribes you a pill, this doesn't mean that it has been approved as being effective and safe for your condition. Many doctors prescribe medicines for 'off-label' use, which means that they have been officially approved for use in other types of conditions, not the one that they are being prescribed for in this particular instance. What this means is that their use in this area has not been rigorously studied or approved by regulatory agencies. Patients are not always told when they are being prescribed a drug off-label. So you may want to ask: 'Is this medicine approved for my condition or is this an off-label use?'

Even when there is reliable evidence to show that a treatment is effective, this does not necessarily mean it will work for you in your particular situation. Often the people taking part in clinical trials testing the effects of treatments are not representative of the broader population. They tend to be younger and healthier than the people likely to have the treatment in the real world. So it's fair to assume that many treatments will not be as effective for you as they have been in trials. Many other variables can also affect the likelihood that a treatment will help. Studies may, for example, show that a type of surgery is an effective treatment. But whether this is more broadly relevant to you may depend on the skills of your particular surgeon and surgical team, as well as the standards of the facilities and care at the particular hospital where you are having treatment.

And, as one of the Monty Python team once quipped, we are all individuals. Two people with the same health problem may respond quite differently to the same treatment. Your genetic make-up, gender, environment and ethnic background may all affect how you respond to any given treatment. For example, as discussed in the third example, it can't be assumed that treatments for heart disease will work the same way in women as they do in men. This really reinforces the importance of asking, when a treatment is being recommended: 'How well might this treatment work for me in my particular situation?'

EXAMPLE 1
Alarm over antioxidants

These days, it seems you can't go into a chemist or supermarket, or open a magazine or newspaper, without coming across products or advertisements spruiking the benefits of

Believing the marketing hype might make you sick

antioxidants. This is the name given to a group of vitamins and vitamin-like substances that can counteract the effects of a potentially damaging process called oxidation. Including vitamins A, C, E and betacarotene, it's claimed that antioxidants prevent everything from heart disease to cancer and the effects of ageing. Doctors, celebrities and scientists have been enthusiastic in touting their wonders. And of course their manufacturers have too; antioxidants are a multibillion dollar business internationally.

Which just goes to show that believing everything you hear about health products can be dangerous. Millions of people around the world are regularly swallowing antioxidant supplements in the hope they will be good for their health, not realising that they may sometimes actually be harmful.

To be fair, for quite a while it looked like there was real cause for optimism about antioxidants. One of the reasons that fruit and vegetables are thought to be so good for us is that they contain many antioxidants. Laboratory experiments showed that antioxidants tend to counteract the harmful effects of free radicals, which are unstable molecules that can damage cells. Researchers also found that people with high levels of antioxidants in their blood tended to be healthier than those who did not. Studies following large groups of people also found that those who took antioxidant supplements tended to be healthier than those who didn't. But not everyone was convinced by these studies, as they did not rule out the possibility that people who took antioxidants were healthier already, because they also had healthier lifestyles in general. In other words, there was always the possibility that taking antioxidants was simply a sign of having a healthy lifestyle generally, rather than being a cause of good health itself.

It was impossible to be sure that taking antioxidants would be helpful until proper randomised controlled trials were conducted. Chapter 8, 'What is the evidence?', explains more about why randomised controlled trials are important for evaluating the potential benefits and risks involved in any treatment or intervention.

In another reminder of why you can't assume that treatments will be good for you unless they've been carefully evaluated, the tide began to turn on the antioxidant good news story in the mid 1990s. One randomised controlled trial after another threw up the worrying suggestion that not only did antioxidant supplements fail to deliver the health benefits that had been so widely promised, but that they might do harm. Over the past decade or so, many randomised controlled trials and systematic reviews—which assess the results of multiple trials—have found higher death rates amongst people taking antioxidants, especially if taken in high doses.

One recent review estimated that death rates were 5 per cent higher in people taking supplements containing vitamins A, E or betacarotene.[2] The authors thought this was probably an underestimate, and added that they were unable to rule out the possibility that vitamin C supplements also did harm. They noted that their findings applied to synthetic antioxidants so should not discourage people from consuming antioxidants where they occur naturally—in fruit and vegetables. No one has suggested vitamin supplements should be avoided for people with serious nutritional deficiencies; the concern is about their use by normal people, who unfortunately happen to account for the majority of people who take them.

As you might imagine, these findings have not been universally welcomed. They represent a powerful threat to the lucrative markets of many companies, which have since funded skilful public relations and marketing campaigns to continue touting antioxidants. A recent search of the Blackmores website, for example, found many statements extolling the 'benefits' of antioxidants and no mention they might be dangerous. As well, it is only natural that scientific findings challenging accepted wisdoms take time to gain acceptance. The attitudes of many doctors and other health professionals promoting vitamins have been slow to change. Even leading medical journals have continued to publish articles recommending the use of supplements.[3]

So it is not surprising that the message to be wary of antioxidants does not seem to have reached many people. Indeed, one study suggested vitamin use increased in the United States over the past ten years, just as research was emerging to suggest it might be wiser for many people to stop use. It's been estimated that 10 to 20 per cent of adults in North America and Europe—or between 80 and 160 million people—consume dietary supplements, many of which include antioxidants. One study in the United States found that more than half of postmenopausal women were taking antioxidant supplements in some form, at maximum doses and for long periods of time.[4] These researchers estimated that for every million people exposed to toxic combinations or amounts of antioxidant supplements, about 9000 premature deaths could have occurred.

Many people might assume that because vitamin supplements are so easily available and so widely promoted that they must be safe and, further, good for you. It's a dangerous assumption. Millions of people are spending large sums of money on products that are, at best, useless and, at worst, harmful. It's a chilling reminder of the importance of asking tough questions about any type of health treatment or product—even those easily available over-the-counter in any supermarket or pharmacist.

EXAMPLE 2
Managing dementia

As increasing numbers of people live into their ninth and tenth decade or even longer, many of us are dealing with the challenges of dementia in family members. Dementia is a general term used to describe problems arising from changes in or damage to the brain. These changes can have different causes, but in general the risk of someone getting dementia increases as they grow older. For the individual, dementia can signal the beginning of a loss of self-identity and control. Those who care for people with dementia must also grapple with

Too much medicine can be harmful

many confronting issues, including the grief of losing aspects of the person they know, while often having to cope with the difficult and challenging behaviours that can accompany dementia.

How best to manage the burden of dementia is one of the more complex health problems we face, both at an individual level and more broadly as a society. This is partly because dementia becomes more common as people get older, so often those affected are already struggling with other health problems due to ageing. As well as being more likely to have many health problems, older people are much more vulnerable to the side effects of medications. Ironically, at least some of the decline in mental functioning seen as people get older is due to the side effects of commonly used medications.[5]

The vulnerability of the elderly to side effects means it is even more important to be sure that any treatment is worth the potential risks. Complicating the issue further is the fact that as dementia worsens, people may become unable to be involved in making decisions about their care and treatment. The responsibility for making decisions about treatments can fall on their family members or other carers.

This brings us to another reason why dealing with dementia is such a complex issue: often it has implications for the health and well-being of people other than the person with dementia. Carers are not only vulnerable to distress and exhaustion but their own physical health can suffer too. Good care for people with dementia often relies upon there being good support for their carers.

You can understand from all this background why good dementia care means taking a holistic approach to meeting the many needs of patients, their families and carers. It means so much more than prescribing a pill. But you can no doubt also understand why people might hope for a 'miracle cure', or believe that it is worth trying a new medicine in the hope that it may make a difference, however small. Yet history has shown the dangers of such an approach. Many of the treatments for dementia, which were at first heralded as promising breakthroughs, have turned out to be much less effective than first hoped. Even worse, they have often also been found to be harmful, and sometimes outright deadly, when used in such a vulnerable group as the elderly.

There is a long history of prescribing antipsychotic drugs and tranquillisers to patients with dementia, particularly those in nursing homes, in an attempt to control some of the difficult behaviours associated with the condition. However, numerous reports have warned that these drugs are of only modest benefit while simultaneously involving a risk of serious complications. Such concerns led to tighter controls on the use of older types of antipsychotic drugs in nursing homes.

As newer antipsychotic medicines have become available in recent years, it was hoped these would be more effective and safer. However, there is mounting evidence that they are neither more effective, nor safer. There are grave concerns about their potential to cause serious side effects, such as strokes. Although health authorities in several countries have issued formal warnings about the risks of these drugs for people with dementia, they continue to be extremely widely used, as illustrated by the studies described below.

One study found that in 2000–2001, antipsychotic drugs were being taken by just over one-quarter of all patients in United States nursing homes who received Medicare benefits. Most were taking the newer types of antipsychotic drugs and were not being given the drugs in accordance with prescribing guidelines, many receiving worryingly high doses.[6] In other words, these findings suggest that many people with dementia are being exposed to the risk of serious side effects, without a high likelihood of benefit. Many other drugs are also widely used in people with dementia despite scant evidence of their benefit, including anticonvulsants, antidepressants and anti-anxiety drugs.

Meanwhile, one of the most hyped developments in dementia treatment in recent years has been the advent of drugs called cholinesterase inhibitors, a well-known example being donepezil, sold under the brand name Aricept. These drugs have been widely described as a 'breakthrough' for their supposed benefits in enhancing mental functioning, and many doctors and carers have reported noticing improvements in patients who take them. However, studies have shown that doctors and carers also often notice improvements in patients taking placebos or 'dummy' pills. It turns out that the more high-quality trials that are done, the less it looks like these drugs will live up to the initial hype. Generally, it seems they are likely to have only a modest benefit. Indeed, the National Institute for Health and Clinical Excellence in the United Kingdom has revised its advice about their use; it no longer recommends them for all people with dementia but says they should be limited to those with moderately severe disease. One recent journal article said it was a tragedy these drugs had turned out to be of such 'marginal benefit'. It also sounded the alarm that the intense focus on them had diverted resources and attention from other approaches to dementia care, such as providing better support for carers and safer environments for people with dementia.[7]

Despite all the hype and hope about drug treatments for dementia, it is generally advised that non-drug approaches should be tried first. The National Institute for Health and Clinical Excellence recommends the development of tailored care plans, which includes providing carers with training courses and skills in communication and problem-solving. However, when so much attention is focused on drug treatments, it often means that these other approaches—such as psychological therapies, or better training of nursing-home staff or family carers, or adapting the patient's physical environment to their needs—are under-researched and underfunded.

Ensuring patients and their carers receive the help they need means being prepared to ask: 'How well does this treatment work?'—particularly if what is being offered is a drug with only modest benefits and the risk of serious side effects. Dementia is like many other chronic health problems in that it is necessary to keep asking this question throughout the course of the illness. It is not a question that you can afford to ask only once; it has to be asked again and again. The history of dementia is also a reminder of the importance of asking the question already outlined in chapter 4: 'What are my options?' Asking both of these questions at every stage of the dementia journey may help make for a smoother, safer ride.

EXAMPLE 3
Heart disease

In matters of the heart, men and women really are different. This is true in so many ways, but one of the less obvious ones is that when it comes to

Women and men really are different

heart disease, women cannot assume that the findings from research will be as relevant for them as they are for men. Many treatments have been developed largely on the basis of studies involving men, so assuming that a treatment will work as effectively in women as it does in men can be a mistake. The history of heart disease treatments is a reminder of the importance of asking: 'How well will this treatment work for me?'

It is also a reminder that generalisations about how people will experience a health problem or respond to a treatment can be misleading. Heart disease, for example, develops quite differently in women than it does in men because of differences in our biology and behaviour. As a result, women are generally some years older than men when they first suffer problems such as heart attacks. This is probably one of the reasons why heart disease has often been seen as a 'man's problem'—because men tend to be affected younger.

This perception of heart disease as a male problem may also help explain why health services tend to treat women quite differently to men when it comes to heart disease. Women are less likely, for example, to be referred for potentially life-saving treatments, whether blood-thinning medications, surgery or procedures to clear blocked arteries.

This may happen because health services are sometimes less likely to be proactive at treating patients who are older. As well, some of these treatments may be less effective in women. Women are more likely to suffer complications from bypass surgery, for example, perhaps because they tend to have smaller coronary arteries, which can make surgery more difficult. Another possibility is that women may be more vulnerable to side effects of various treatments because they tend to be older when they need care for heart disease. Studies in different countries have also shown that women are less likely to be referred to cardiac rehabilitation programs, which support patients in making healthy lifestyle changes and managing their illness more effectively.

For all of these reasons, women with heart disease don't tend to do as well as men. This is not only because they are generally older (and thus also more likely to have other health problems, such as diabetes) because even after taking such factors into account, they are still less likely to survive a heart attack or other cardiovascular complication. Clearly, women with heart disease have good cause for asking plenty of careful questions of their doctors.

Even when hospitals make real efforts to improve the care of patients with heart disease by encouraging the use of standard treatment guidelines and ensuring good planning when patients are discharged from hospital, research has shown that these measures are less likely to be applied to women.[8]

Another reason for women's inferior care and survival rates is that they may have different symptoms than men when having a heart attack or angina. While men often present with chest pain, women are more likely to have nausea, vomiting and neck, back or jaw pain. This is thought to be one reason why they are also more likely to delay seeking treatment as they may be less likely to recognise their symptoms as a potential heart warning, and so may their doctors when they do eventually seek help.

Perhaps one of the most important reasons for women's poorer outcomes is because so much of the research into heart disease has been based on men. This is not just true of heart disease, though. Before 1985, women were rarely included in clinical trials at all, partly because the thalidomide disaster in the 1960s had made researchers wary of exposing women (and potentially their unborn children) to new drugs. As well, male physiology was traditionally considered the standard by which to judge new treatments.

This meant that the implications for women from clinical trials were not always clear. Just because a treatment worked in men—or didn't—did not mean that it would have the same effect in women. As a result of such concerns, the Food and Drug Administration and the National Institutes of Health in the United States ruled in 1993 that women and minority groups must be included in clinical trials.

While more women are now included in trials of heart disease treatments, it remains the case that what is known about many treatments and the nature of heart disease is based upon how it occurs in men, and cannot be assumed to always apply to women. It also suggests that women who are being given information about tests or treatments for heart disease should make very sure that the information is relevant to them.

For example, guidelines widely recommend the use of ACE inhibitor drugs, such as Capoten and Prinivil, and cholesterol-lowering drugs called statins, such as Zocor and Lipitor, in people with heart disease. But it is not clear whether they are likely to be as helpful for women as men. One review of studies testing the use of ACE inhibitors in patients who'd just had a heart attack couldn't show that they made any difference for women. This could mean that the drugs aren't as effective in women, or it could also simply reflect that so few women were included in the trials that there weren't enough to measure any impact.

Similarly, there has been considerable controversy over whether statins are as effective in women as they are in men. In the major trials testing these drugs, women have generally accounted for no more than one in five participants. How widely statins should be prescribed to women is not clear as a result, with some experts saying there is not enough evidence to warrant their widespread use, while others recommending use by women with many risk factors for cardiovascular disease.[9] It is remarkable, given this debate, that some Australian research suggests women are actually more likely than men to be prescribed statins.[10]

What all of this means is that it is particularly important for women to ask their doctors about how well a treatment is likely to work for them. Assuming that a treatment will work as effectively in women as it does in men can be a mistake, and this lesson should also be considered more broadly. Many people, perhaps because of their health, age or ethnic background, will find that the results of trials may not be relevant to their situation. Everyone needs to ask the question: 'Are there any reasons to think that this treatment will not work for me in my situation?'

Conclusion

How well does that treatment work?

While the last example focuses on the particular issue of women and heart disease, it raises a much broader point.

Even when treatments have been proven to be effective in large studies, this does not necessarily mean they will work for you in your situation. You need to know more than 'How well does this treatment work?'—you need to know: 'How well might this treatment work for me, in my situation?'

Unfortunately, you cannot always rely on health professionals to be able to answer this question as fully as you might like. They may not have the time, inclination or expertise to hunt out the information needed to give a full response. If you are having difficulty getting these questions answered, you have a few options. You could find another health professional. Or you could track down alternative sources of information. (We have listed some reliable sources of health information at the back of this book.) Health services and health organisations generally are becoming much more proactive at providing information to help patients and health professionals assess the merits of various treatment options.

Of course, there is not always the opportunity or time to ask questions about how well a treatment works. Increasingly, however, many of the most common health problems are chronic conditions such as arthritis and diabetes, involving ongoing treatment over a long period of time. It is with these chronic conditions that people have the most to gain from asking: 'How well might this treatment work for me, in my situation?'

More questions about treatments

How well does that treatment work?

- How many people need to take this treatment in order for one person to benefit?

- How well might this treatment work for me, in my situation?

- How long will it take for this treatment to have a useful effect?

- Is this treatment approved for my condition?

- Are there any other treatment options, which don't involve taking pills?

Six

What are the side effects?

Every day, thousands of people around the world are inadvertently harmed by the health care that was meant to help them. Side effects from medicines and complications from operations are far more common than many people realise. You can't always rely on doctors or other health professionals to tell you about the risks of medicines or other treatments. You must ask what these risks are, how likely they are to occur, and how they might be expected to affect you, in your personal situation. You might also want to ask what to do if side effects occur: should you, for example, stop the medicine, lower the dose, or see a doctor immediately? It is particularly important for older people to ask these questions, as they are at greatest risk of suffering complications from health care.

After a terrible car accident, a woman known to us only as Mrs Ong spent three months in hospital, unable to move because of a badly fractured pelvis. Because of her high risk of developing a blood clot, she was put on a blood-thinning medicine called warfarin as a preventative measure. This should have been stopped as soon as Mrs Ong was able to walk again, but a series of errors and misunderstandings between the doctors involved in her care meant that it continued to be prescribed after she left hospital.

Some months later, Mrs Ong died from a massive stroke caused by an interaction between the blood-thinning drug and some antibiotics which had been prescribed for an infection. Mrs Ong's relatives were told the stroke was probably due to the blood-thinning medicine, but were not told that she did not need to be taking the drug in the first place or that a well-known drug interaction had been involved. A coroner was told that Mrs Ong had suffered the stroke as a result of blood abnormalities following a car accident, and on this basis concluded that he did not have an interest in the case.

This tragic story has been put on the public record by experts working to improve the safety of health care because it raises so many important issues for anyone coming into contact with health services.[1] It shows how easily things can go wrong once people enter the health system, especially when multiple doctors are involved in their care, and how patients and their families often are not well informed about the potential harms of their care—even after these have occurred.

It is also a reminder of the importance of asking about the possible side effects and interactions of any medicine, whether it is prescribed by a doctor, bought from a supermarket or dispensed by a naturopath. The potential for serious interactions to result when warfarin and antibiotics are mixed is well documented. One can only wonder how differently things might have turned out if Mrs Ong or her family had known to ask about her medicine, whether she needed to keep taking it, and what were the potential side effects and interactions to watch out for.

While Mrs Ong's death was a tragedy, what makes it even worse is that her story is not as unusual as you'd expect. Making such a claim even twenty years ago would have brought angry denials from the medical industry. These days, however, few can argue with the truth of such a statement. So many studies in so many countries have documented the dangers of modern health care.

You may have heard of the saying that 'every system is perfectly designed to produce the results that it gets'. In other words, if a system is getting bad results, it is because that is the inevitable result of its bad design. The sad reality is that our complex, fragmented health systems make it very difficult to ensure patients will receive safe care, especially in institutions like hospitals. If you or someone you love is going into hospital, the third example in this chapter shows the importance of being as informed as possible about all aspects of the care. This may help reduce the chance of things going wrong.

As Mrs Ong's case illustrates, when patients are harmed it is often because there have been multiple errors and communication lapses. It is all too easy for such breakdowns to occur when the trend towards subspecialisation often means that several doctors are involved in a patient's care, sometimes without any one of them taking overall responsibility for the totality of that care. The end result of these breakdowns in care may be something as common as a wound infection or as catastrophic as surgery being conducted on the wrong body part—or wrong patient.

But the majority of harms caused by modern health care involve medicines. It might be because the wrong drug or the wrong dose has been prescribed or taken, or because of side effects or

Harms of medicines are downplayed

interactions with other drugs—which may or may not have been predictable. At the same time that the benefits of medicines and other treatments are often overstated, the potential harms are often understated. The most common sources of information about medicines—the media, health professionals, clinical trials, drug advertisements and marketing—are all known to downplay the potential harms.

Many people make the mistake of assuming that because a drug or a complementary health product is available and on the market that it must be safe. This is a mistake that can prove fatal. No drug or treatment is free of the risk of side effects. In Australia alone, it has been estimated that almost 2 million people suffer some sort of harm related to medicines each year, with about 138 000 suffering such serious problems that they require hospitalisation. Most of these harms are caused by side effects.[2] In the United States, it has been estimated that problems caused by medicines are the fifth most common cause of death after heart disease, cancer, stroke and lung disease.[3] In the United Kingdom, it is thought that 250 000 people are admitted to hospital every year because of problems related to medicines.[4]

Even cough medicines, so easily and widely available, can involve life-threatening risks. In the United States, health authorities have called for caution in the use of cough medicines in children under two after they were blamed for the deaths of three babies in 2005. The Centers for Disease Control and Prevention estimates that more than 1500 children under age two were treated for problems related to the use of these medicines in the US in 2004–05. Such side effects are particularly alarming, given that these medicines are unlikely to have any benefits for young children.[5]

It is not easy to predict or establish the side effects of medicines: people taking medicines tend to have various health conditions and, when a problem arises, it can be difficult to be sure whether it is related to the medicine or their underlying health problem. If a side effect is uncommon, it may only become apparent after hundreds of thousands of people have taken a medicine. It is not unusual for side effects to be discovered years after a drug has been on the market. Agencies which regulate the approval of drugs, such as the Food and Drug Administration in the United States, have been widely criticised for failing to adequately protect public safety in this regard.[6] Nor can you rely on drug companies to be open and frank about their products: there have been too many examples of drug companies covering up information about drugs' harms.

This is one of the reasons that drug safety experts advise doctors and patients to be cautious about using new drugs. Often they are no more effective than existing drugs, while the true picture about their safety is still unknown. As is shown by the first example in this chapter on arthritis, premature enthusiasm for new drugs can have deadly consequences. Even when the side effects of medications are well understood, you can't be sure that you or your doctor will be told about them.

The product information, which guides the use of drugs, is often out of date and can contain potentially harmful recommendations, according to an evaluation of the Australian product information for medicines used to treat thyroid disease.[7] The implications of this study are worrying— not only for the 200 000 or so Australians taking thyroid medicines, but for anyone relying on product information for advice about the safe use of drugs. (The information used in consumer medicine information leaflets is also usually based on the product information.)

All of these issues are particularly relevant for older people because they are most likely to come to harm in hospitals and are also at greatest risk of suffering side effects from medicines, surgery or other procedures. Sometimes older patients find it more difficult to question their doctors or other health professionals. This reluctance, while understandable, can be a serious health hazard, as illustrated by the second example on caring for older people. They (and their families and carers) have the most to gain from asking their doctor or other health professional: 'What are the potential side effects of this treatment?'

EXAMPLE 1
Arthritis drugs scandal

'Wonder' drugs can be a health hazard

In June 2000, then Australian Minister for Health, Dr Michael Wooldridge issued a most extraordinary media statement. In it he announced that the first of a new class of arthritis drugs called COX-2 inhibitors would be funded by the Australian government. He said the drug, celecoxib (sold under the brand name Celebrex), was significantly safer than older types of drugs used to treat arthritis and called it a 'major breakthrough in arthritis therapy'.[8]

It was highly unusual that a health minister would feel the need to single out any one drug for such an enthusiastic plug. It was even more remarkable considering that a careful reading of the scientific literature would have shown there were already rumblings of concern about the safety of COX-2 inhibitors. Over the next few years, these rumblings turned into a roar of alarm and an international scandal damaging public trust in drug regulatory agencies, medical journals and drug companies alike.

We now know that tens of thousands of people around the world paid a very high price—suffering heart attacks and strokes—for following advice to take drugs that they had been assured, wrongly as it turned out, were safer than older types of arthritis drugs. Taxpayers and patients also paid a very high price for the overly enthusiastic promotion of these drugs, which reaped huge profits for their manufacturers. While safety concerns surround many of the COX-2 inhibitors, including the one so warmly endorsed by Dr Wooldridge, the most alarming case was that of rofecoxib, which was sold under the brand name Vioxx by the drug giant Merck.

The history of rofecoxib reveals that many different groups failed to protect the public's safety. The Food and Drug Administration in the United States was slow to act on evidence that rofecoxib was associated with an increased risk of heart attacks and strokes. One of the world's leading medical journals, the *New England Journal of Medicine*, was slow to publish corrections to a study that had minimised concerns about a heart disease risk. The drug's manufacturer, Merck, suppressed studies raising the alarm about rofecoxib's safety, and also instructed its sales representatives to downplay such concerns, while giving them misleading information to use in their sales pitches to doctors.[9]

The drug was not withdrawn from the market until 2004 although concerns about its potential to cause cardiovascular problems were raised in 1998, before it had even been approved for marketing, and were reinforced by a major study published in 2000. Meanwhile, the media was overly quick to trumpet the virtues of COX-2 inhibitors.

As a result of such delays, cover-ups and misleading promotions, millions more people were exposed to the risk of side effects from rofecoxib than should have been. By the time rofecoxib was taken off the market, it had been prescribed to more than 20 million people around the world. More than 100 million prescriptions had been filled in the United States alone, while in Australia it accounted for 40 per cent of spending on non-steroidal anti-inflammatory drugs.[10] Meanwhile, safety concerns have continued to dog other COX-2 inhibitors. In late 2007, for instance, the drug Prexige was withdrawn from the Australian market because of serious liver damage associated with its use. At the time of its recall, the National Prescribing Service cautioned that side effects from medicines are a big problem more broadly, especially given that a staggering 70 per cent of Australians are taking a medicine of some sort—whether prescription or non-prescription—at any one time.

The COX-2 disaster led to a major inquiry into the Food and Drug Administration in the United States, and wide-ranging recommendations for improving drug safety. But this is far from the only drug safety scandal of recent years. In 2007, Purdue Pharma, manufacturer of the painkiller oxycodone (sold under the brand name OxyContin), pleaded guilty to falsely marketing the drug in a way that played down its addictive properties and led to scores of people becoming addicted.[11] Meanwhile, GlaxoSmithKline has also been accused of playing down safety concerns surrounding a diabetes drug, Avandia, which has been linked to an increased risk of heart attacks and has been taken by about 7 million people internationally.[12] Bayer also suppressed information about the dangers of its drug aprotinin, which was widely used to reduce bleeding in patients undergoing heart surgery, and also hid unfavourable data on its cholesterol-lowering drug, cerivastatin, before it was taken off the market in 2001.[13] And there are plenty more examples of drug companies engaging in misleading practices.

What makes the COX-2 story so special, however, is that these drugs were developed and promoted for their safety. It's a powerful reminder of the need to be sceptical whenever anyone is promoting a new drug—whether the 'breakthrough' promise is being made by a health minister, a professor or a TV advertisement. Too often when someone claims a new drug is a 'breakthrough', what this really means is that only time will tell whether it is as useful or as safe as is being claimed. Even when a drug has been around for years, it's important to ask questions about its side effects, including: 'What is known about the side effects of this treatment?' and 'How likely are these side effects to occur?' and 'How might they affect me, in my situation?' You could also ask: 'Are there any non-drug treatments that I could have instead of a medicine?'

When patients develop problems that are thought to be related to their medicines, health professionals are encouraged to report these to regulatory authorities, so that potential side-effect problems can be identified and studied. Traditionally, patients have not been encouraged to be involved in this process, which means an important source of information about side effects has been neglected. If you do develop problems that may be related to your medication, it's worth asking your doctor or pharmacist whether these should be reported to the appropriate regulatory authority.

EXAMPLE 2
Caring for older people

It is especially wise to ask questions

Sarah Jones (not her real name) wasn't at all happy when she came home with a sample of pills that her GP had been given by a drug company sales representative. The GP had suggested Sarah try the pills in the hope they might reduce her risk of suffering another painful fracture of the vertebrae in her back. The GP reassured Sarah about the drug's safety, perhaps because she knew that Sarah didn't really like taking medicines unless they were absolutely necessary. Don't worry, this drug is perfectly safe, the doctor told Sarah.

However, Sarah was not convinced. She rang a friend who did a quick search on the Internet and found a reputable site—the National Institute for Health and Clinical Excellence in the United Kingdom—which made it clear that this drug, like many of those prescribed to prevent bone fractures associated with osteoporosis, was known to have a number of potential side effects, some serious.

Sarah decided against taking the drug. The way she saw it, the potential for side effects outweighed the potential for benefits—especially as she was well into her nineties and knew from experience that she was particularly susceptible to suffering problems from medicines because of her age and physical frailty. Sarah had previously become quite unwell after being prescribed amiodarone for an abnormal heart rhythm. Later she learned that a number of studies had raised serious concerns about this drug's safety.[14]

In many ways, Sarah's case symbolises one of the big dilemmas confronting modern medicine. As the population lives longer and longer, more and more elderly people are seeking treatment for ongoing health problems. Many end up taking multiple medications over long periods of time. But they are particularly vulnerable to side effects because of their reduced body weight, poorer health and other factors related to growing older. Often there is uncertainty about the benefits of medicines in the elderly, as they tend to be excluded from clinical trials testing new drugs. The result is that many older people are at significant risk of being harmed by medicines, and often for uncertain gain. In the worst case scenario, many end up being prescribed one medicine to counteract the side effects of another one. Some experts have argued that illness caused by medications is a critical health issue and 'the most significant treatable geriatric health problem'.[15]

Many studies have documented the extent of the problem. For instance, when Australian researchers investigated unplanned admissions to Royal Hobart Hospital involving patients aged seventy-five and older, they found 30 per cent may have been due to a medicine-related complication.[16] Just over half of these cases were considered to have been preventable. Meanwhile, a large study of Australian veterans found that one-fifth of those aged over seventy were dispensed at least one potentially inappropriate medicine in the first half of 2005.[17] On the basis of these findings, the researchers estimated that every six months almost 400000 Australians aged seventy or over are given a potentially inappropriate medicine.

To be fair, however, it is important to point out that such studies generally document only the harms that are being caused by medicines, without giving the other side of the equation. Doctors point out that there is now reliable evidence that treating a range of conditions in the elderly does more good than harm, on average. Some patients may develop serious side effects but a larger number have their lives prolonged. Nonetheless, the increasing use of medicines in the elderly means that more older people are suffering side effects, and therefore need to know what questions to ask their doctors about these problems.

Between 1981 and 2002, there was a fivefold increase in the rate of older patients being admitted to Western Australian hospitals because of problems caused by medicines.[18] The biggest increases were in those aged eighty or older. The medicines most often involved were those prescribed for cardiovascular diseases, especially blood-thinning drugs. The researchers estimated that, on the basis of their findings, about one-third of people would require hospital treatment for an adverse drug reaction at some time in their lives between the ages of sixty and eighty-five. The researchers noted that experts in the United States had identified forty-eight classes of medication that should not be given to the elderly. One of the reasons for drawing up this list was their concern about the rising costs of having to treat drug complications.

A worrying aspect of these findings is that many people may not realise their problems are due to their medicines, as this is often only discovered if a formal study or review is undertaken. One Australian study of older people considered at high risk of medication misadventure found that one-fifth had experienced such a problem which had not been detected in routine care.[19]

The risk of patients suffering harm from medicines can be reduced by what are called medication reviews. This involves the treating doctor, pharmacist and patient themselves critically examining all of the medications being taken by the patient. However, such reviews are not nearly as widely available as they should be. One expert has estimated that medication reviews are conducted for only about one in ten people likely to benefit from them.[20]

The message seems loud and clear. The elderly—and those who care for them—have much to gain from asking questions about the potential for any treatment to cause harms such as side effects. The simple question—'Can I have a medication review?'—could be life-saving.

Older people are not only more susceptible to harms from medicines: it is hard to think of any treatment or procedure, whether mainstream or complementary, which will not involve more risks for an older person. They are, for example, at increased risk of things going wrong when in hospital, as outlined in the next example. In a landmark study of adverse events occurring in Australian hospitals, three-quarters of all preventable deaths occurred in patients over sixty-five. This age group was ten times more likely to die from an adverse event in hospital than patients under forty-five.[21]

EXAMPLE 3
Avoiding harm in hospitals

Constant vigilance is needed Jessica Santillan, the daughter of a truck driver in Mexico, was born with a heart condition that left her extremely breathless and weak. If she attempted any physical exertion, she inevitably fainted. Her only hope for a normal life was to have a heart-lung transplant. Her family begged in the streets to raise money to send her to the United States for the operation. Amazingly, their dreams came true after their fundraising campaign won the support of an American businessman. In February 2003, Jessica's father brought her to Duke University Medical Center in North Carolina.

There a terrible mistake occurred. Jessica, seventeen, was transplanted with incompatible organs, and died a few weeks later. After conducting a thorough investigation, the hospital made a full confession of its mistakes and changed its procedures to reduce the risks of such errors happening again.[22]

For Jessica's family, the tragedy of her loss must have been made even worse by the betrayal of the faith they had put in modern medicine. Her death is a poignant reminder of the high stakes of health care. While modern medicine, with all its sophisticated technology and knowledge, can achieve so much more than once would have been thought possible, it also has an ever-increasing potential to do serious damage. In a sense, modern medicine is caught in a catch-22: patients who once would have been judged too sick or too old to have any medical intervention are now undergoing complicated surgery or having other treatments. They are therefore more vulnerable to any problems arising out of such treatments.

The combination of the increasing vulnerability of patients with the uncertainty of modern medicine and the poor design of health-care systems means that it is all too easy for things to go wrong, especially in hospitals. More people die as a result of problems with their health care than in road accidents, and it is often said that it is safer to travel by aeroplane than go to hospital. Indeed, it's estimated that the number of people dying because of their health care in the United States is equivalent to two jumbo jets full of passengers crashing every three days. Studies around the world have found that between 7.5 per cent and 12.9 per cent of hospital admissions are associated with adverse events, such as medication errors, surgical complications or infections picked up in hospital.[23]

It is not only the physical harm caused by such problems that is a concern. When people put their lives into the hands of others, it is a profound act of trust. When this trust is breached, it can leave a deep emotional scar. Doctors and other health professionals know that things can go wrong, even with the best of care and intentions. But patients do not always realise this, and people who've been the victims of hospital misadventures can struggle to come to terms with what has happened to them or their loved ones.

Often such problems are reported in the media as if they are all due to medical negligence or 'bad' health professionals. In reality, medical negligence or malpractice is to blame for only a small proportion of the problems that occur in hospitals or other health services. Most problems result from the way systems are set up and run, such as inadequately trained or supervised staff, bad rostering, and poor communication and follow-up systems. In some ways, this means it is much harder to prevent such problems than if the solution lay in simply weeding out the incompetent doctors.

It also is a reminder of the need for constant vigilance. It is not enough to know that you have a good doctor whom you trust. Things can go wrong no matter how competent or well-meaning the health professionals who are looking after you. Because of this, many hospitals and health services around the world are making strenuous efforts to make care safer. One way they are doing this is asking that patients, their families and carers ensure they are as informed as possible. The Australian Commission on Safety and Quality in Health Care published some tips for what patients, their families and carers can do to reduce the risk of things going wrong.[24] The main message is the importance of asking questions, including about the risks of any treatment. You could also ask: 'Could my symptoms be due to side effects or a complication of treatment?'

Conclusion
What are the side effects?

Side effects and other complications from health care and medications are all too common. Not all of these are preventable—sometimes things will go wrong, no matter what. But it is generally agreed that it should be possible to prevent as many as half of such complications.

Sometimes your need for care may be so urgent that there is no chance to consider issues such as side effects. But often there is time and opportunity to ask these questions. This is especially important as more and more people are seeking help for chronic conditions, which often involve long-term treatment. And it is especially important to ask these questions given the increasing number of older people seeking treatment. The trend towards using medicines in preventing illness or treating so-called lifestyle problems is also another reason to be cautious. If a treatment is not life-saving, there may be less reason to risk side effects.

The point is not that any treatment should be rejected simply because it has side effects. There are few, if any, treatments which are completely free of risk. It may be worth having a treatment which is likely to cause unpleasant side effects (such as chemotherapy, for example) if it is potentially life-saving. And it's a mistake to assume that so-called 'natural' health products are harmless. Many problems have arisen out of the use of complementary medicines and practices. And, as already discussed in chapter 5, 'How well does that treatment work?', even vitamins or other products that are widely available in supermarkets and chemists may have a downside.[25]

The point is to make sure you understand the potential side effects of any treatment, how likely these are, how they may affect you in your personal situation, and what you should do if they occur. You need this information to be able to weigh up whether the potential benefits of treatment outweigh any potential side effects or other harms. Each person will weigh up these factors differently. A side effect that some people consider unimportant may be judged as unacceptable by others. The likelihood of side effects and their importance may vary according to where you live, your age, your physical health, your lifestyle and your priorities. Your ethnic and cultural background may also influence your susceptibility to side effects; some ethnic groups such as those from Asia, may, for example, be more likely to suffer side effects from cardiovascular medicines.[26]

Asking basic questions about the potential side effects of a treatment may lead you in other directions. Many heart attacks might have been prevented if patients seeking relief from arthritis had decided to try non-drug solutions—such as exercises or losing weight—instead of taking medications like COX-2 inhibitors.

More questions about side effects

What are the side effects?

- What is known about the side effects of this treatment?
- How likely are these side effects to occur?
- How might they affect me, in my situation?
- What should I do if side effects occur?
- Could my symptoms be due to side effects or a complication of treatment?
- Will this medicine interact with the other products I'm taking?
- What can I do to reduce the risk of side effects or other complications?
- Is consumer medicines information available about this product?
- Are there any non-drug treatments that I could have instead of a medicine?
- Should I have a medication review?

Seven

Will this operation really help?

While surgical operations and high-tech procedures can be life-saving, they can also be deadly. Many commonly performed operations and procedures have been poorly tested and some remain unproven—which means we do not know their true benefits and harms. In the first example in this chapter we discover there is little good evidence for a common shoulder operation, and in the second example there is no high-quality evidence to support a popular procedure which involves injecting bone cement into the spine. The third example looks at the pros and cons of caesarean section versus vaginal birth, and again we see the value of a 'decision aid'. Asking questions before you go under the knife might save your life.

Brian Moynihan had recently turned seventy, but was still as fit as an ox. Starting his working life as a carpenter at age thirteen, he'd gone on to build everything from tables and chairs, to houses and skyscrapers.[1] Moving from the city to the country in his sixties, organic gardening had become a serious passion, with all the intense physical exertion that it can involve. After some particularly strenuous excavation, involving digging in a very awkward position over several days, Brian tried to lift a load that was just that little bit too heavy. Excruciating pain shot through his shoulder, and he lost almost all power and movement in his right arm. Diagnosed in the weeks following the incident with what was described as a 'rotator cuff tear', shoulder surgery was recommended and a date for the operation was set.

As many readers would already know, disabling shoulder pain is extremely common, often brought on by heavy lifting or repetitive movements in awkward positions. Treatments include rest, physiotherapy, painkillers and the more serious option of surgery under general anaesthetic, which is sometimes recommended. But believe it or not, most of these widely used treatments have been very poorly tested, making it extremely difficult to know which are best and how much they might help you.

The gold standard for evaluating how well a treatment works—whether that treatment is a drug, physiotherapy, or an operation—is a randomised controlled trial. This is where a large group of patients is randomly divided into two equal-sized groups; one group has the treatment being evaluated and the other group has another treatment, or no treatment. For shoulder surgery, as it happens, there have been only a tiny number of such trials, and in each case the group who had surgery ended up not much better off than the group who didn't have it. That doesn't mean that no one benefits from surgery, it just means it has not yet been very well evaluated.

After asking a GP and a surgeon a lot of questions about the pros and cons of the operation, taking a looking at what scientific evidence he could find, and discussing it with his family and friends, Brian decided not to have surgery and instead try to let his shoulder heal naturally. Though virtually useless at the beginning, the power and range of movement in his arm slowly improved, and a year or so down the track it is almost as good as it was before. Brian is back digging, gardening, performing in theatre productions and doing the odd bit of building, too.

Mrs Green was not so lucky. A mother of two teenage children, she suffered a rotator cuff injury while playing tennis. Two surgeons recommended physiotherapy and strengthening exercises but, frustrated by her inability to garden, she consulted a third surgeon, who agreed to operate while pointing out that it was not strongly recommended. As a result of complications during surgery, she suffered a brain injury that left her in a vegetative state for the rest of her life. While all surgery carries risks, and shoulder surgery is not unusually risky, Mrs Green's experience serves as a tragic example of the danger of undergoing an operation than could well have been avoided. Asking questions can't prevent complications happening, but checking whether you really need that operation may be a very good move.[2]

After scandals like thalidomide, nowadays there are legal requirements that prescription drugs be tested in randomised controlled trials before they are allowed onto the market. These trials may now be mandatory, but they are still sometimes poorly done or heavily influenced by pharmaceutical company sponsors trying to get the answers they want. And while these trials won't always pick up every side effect, particularly rare or long-term ones, at least they have to be done. With operations and procedures, this is not the case: it is a scary fact that new surgical techniques or procedures using the latest technologies can be introduced without the need for rigorous testing in randomised controlled trials. Surgeons tend to 'discover' a new technique or procedure and, after some preliminary evaluation, start promoting it—sometimes with the strong support of manufacturers who benefit from selling the required devices. What this means is that we are often in the dark about how these new techniques and procedures compare to less invasive treatments, or how they compare to doing nothing and letting nature take its course. As we will see, some commonly used operations have been very poorly tested, and some popular procedures have not been tested at all. Asking 'How well has this operation or procedure been tested?' may cause your surgeon some discomfort, but the answer could help you make important decisions.

The first example in this chapter further explores the fact that surgery for shoulder problems has been very poorly evaluated, and until very recently there were no randomised controlled trials comparing surgery to other less invasive treatments like physiotherapy, rest or medications.

The second example examines a procedure where bone cement is injected into vertebrae ('vertebroplasty'), increasingly being used to treat the sharp pain of fractured vertebrae in a person's back, an issue which becomes more common as we age. Promoters of the treatment argue that it's a safe and effective medical breakthrough, but others point out that at this stage it's unproven—there has not been one randomised controlled trial done so far, which means we really don't know its true benefits and harms. Because the pain from these fractures tends to subside over time without any treatment, the concern is that some people may be undergoing this procedure unnecessarily. There are suggestions it could increase the risk of more fractures, so while for some people it provides great immediate pain relief, in the longer run it may be causing more harm than good. Until it is properly tested in high-quality trials, and those trials have produced meaningful results, we simply won't know.

Asking questions and looking for answers can help weigh up risks and benefits

Assessing the benefits and harms of different procedures is always tricky, but when it comes to childbirth, everything seems more complicated. With caesarean births now accounting for more than 20 per cent of all births in many countries, an increasing number of women are now weighing up the pros and cons of caesarean versus vaginal birth.[3] Until very recently it has been hard to find good, easy-to-read information to help make a decision like this—but things are changing. As discussed in chapter 4, 'What are my options?' and elsewhere, information tools called 'decision aids' can sometimes be very helpful, whether in the form of written materials or electronically via the web. As we will see in the third example, recent research suggests that decision aids can address many of the questions and concerns that pregnant women have when deciding which sort of delivery to choose. Women using decision aids end up with greater knowledge, and feel less anxious about their decisions, compared to women not using them. Even with the help of decision aids, these birthing decisions can still be tricky for pregnant women and their families. But at least they are more informed. It's pretty clear that there is one question that more and more people will be asking in the years to come: 'Is there a decision aid available for this operation or procedure?'

EXAMPLE 1
Shoulder surgery

In the late 1990s, an international team of researchers meticulously searched the world's scientific literature for all the studies of treatments for shoulder pain.[4] This process, called a 'systematic review', tends to produce a very reliable form of evidence because it summarises the best studies around. The researchers were looking specifically for randomised controlled trials as these tend to give the most trustworthy results. They found quite a few studies testing medications and physiotherapy, but there were so many variations in the way those trials had been run that it was very difficult to compare the different

Some operations are poorly tested

treatments. It was a bit like comparing apples and oranges. Summarising as best they could, they came up with findings that were not particularly good news for anyone with bad shoulder pain. After reviewing all the studies, the Australian-led team of researchers concluded: 'We could not draw firm conclusions about the efficacy of any of the common interventions currently being used to treat painful shoulders.' While they managed to find thirty-one randomised controlled trials to include in their systematic review of the evidence, not one of those trials compared surgery with other treatments.

A few years later, a team of researchers based in Brazil undertook a similar systematic review—though this time they specifically looked for studies of treatments for the agonising 'rotator cuff tears', like the one Brian experienced after strenuous digging in his garden. In 2004, the Brazilian team published the results of their systematic review.[5] Again, they found no randomised controlled trials comparing surgery to other treatments like physiotherapy or drugs. They concluded there is 'little evidence to support or refute the efficacy of common interventions for tears of the rotator cuff'. This didn't mean that surgery didn't work, it simply meant it hadn't been properly tested.

By 2008, some of those original Australian researchers had gone back to take another look at the scientific studies.[6] This time they found three small trials that compared surgery to other sorts of treatment, involving a total of just over 250 people worldwide. In each of the three trials, it seemed that surgery was no better than the other treatments, causing the researchers to reach similar conclusions as the Brazilians: 'We cannot draw firm conclusions about the effectiveness or safety of surgery for rotator cuff disease.'

All of these systematic reviews of the evidence about how to treat shoulder pain were conducted within the international Cochrane Collaboration, known the world over for its high scientific standards. Like thousands of other systematic reviews, a short summary of the findings are available free at <www.cochrane.org>, which is one of the places it is well worth visiting when deciding whether to undergo an operation or procedure. There are also 'plain language' summaries of these reviews available. (More valuable websites are listed at the end of this book.) Over time, it will become commonplace to ask your doctor or surgeon: 'Have there been any randomised controlled trials?' and 'Is there a systematic review of the evidence available?' The Cochrane Collaboration is one place to get those questions answered.

None of this means there is not a place for surgery in treating shoulder problems—rather it means there is a need for operations to be rigorously tested so people can make informed decisions about whether the potential benefits outweigh the potential harms, and whether to opt for surgery or more 'conservative' treatments like resting, or physiotherapy. In fact, many people believe there is a very important role for surgery, particularly for those with severe shoulder problems for whom other treatments haven't worked. As a team writing in the *British Medical Journal* recently put it: 'For significant persistent disability . . . surgery may be effective at relieving pain and restoring function in patients who have failed conservative treatment.'[7]

EXAMPLE 2
Injecting cement into the spine

Some procedures are unproven

When vertebrae of the spine fracture it can be excruciatingly painful, which is why a procedure called 'vertebroplasty' is becoming increasingly popular. It involves using a needle to inject bone cement into vertebrae, to 'fix' the fracture and stop the fragments of bone from moving and causing intense pain. It's a fairly new procedure but its use is growing, with more than 25 000 being performed in the United States every year.

In Australia, radiologist Dr Bill Clark has done more vertebroplasties than any other doctor.[8] Based out of a private hospital in Sydney, Bill is what's called an 'interventional radiologist', a specialist doctor who uses X-rays and other forms of diagnostic imaging to guide procedures as they actually happen. He and other doctors who perform this procedure are in some way pioneers, reducing people's suffering at one of the new frontiers of medical science.

The problem is that there are no high-quality scientific trials to back up the beliefs of those who promote and perform this procedure. At the time of going to press, there have been no randomised controlled trials completed (two trials are currently underway, but are far from being finished). People do have less pain after the injection, but the long-term risks and benefits are yet to be properly tested. Until those trials are completed, vertebroplasty remains essentially unproven.

'It may be a fantastic treatment,' says Dr Rachelle Buchbinder, 'but let's prove it.'[9] Buchbinder is a professor at Melbourne's Monash University and a doctor specialising in bones and joints (a rheumatologist). She's also a member of the international Cochrane Collaboration with a keen interest in making sure people have the best evidence at their fingertips about how well treatments work. She is concerned when treatments undertaken by her medical colleagues have been poorly tested or not tested at all, and she's become particularly alarmed about vertebroplasty. 'It's unproven,' she says, and for some people 'it may be unnecessary or even harmful'. Motivated initially by a desire to evaluate a potentially promising treatment, Rachelle Buchbinder is running one of the randomised controlled trials of this procedure.

The evidence from early non-randomised trials suggests the procedure can dramatically reduce the pain caused by fracture and can restore full functioning very quickly.[10] However, that pain does tend to resolve naturally over time anyway, and functioning will generally return naturally too. Until proper, high-quality trials are done, it is not clear exactly how well the procedure reduces pain, or returns functioning, compared to doing nothing. It's important to know what the benefits really are in order to weigh them up against the potential harms—which, of course, also remain unknown until the procedure has been properly evaluated.

One of the biggest concerns is that injecting the spine with bone cement may in fact lead to a person suffering more fractures later on, particularly if the cement has leaked into the space between the neighbouring vertebrae. Many people who suffer one fracture in their spine are likely to have another, but Rachelle Buchbinder is worried that the procedure may actually increase that risk of future fracture.

Even promoters of the procedure concede that it may increase the risk of future fracture, although in the view of at least one doctor, contacted for this book, this isn't a problem because future fractures can be repaired in the same way, by injecting bone cement into them. According to that view, one way to prevent more fractures occurring is to inject healthy vertebrae with cement even before they fracture, a practice which is already being undertaken.[11]

Apart from potentially increasing the risk of future fractures, the procedure itself can cause complications—for example, from cement leakage—even when experienced operators are performing the injection. When less experienced doctors are doing the procedure, a patient's chances of having a complication increase. That's because there is often a 'learning curve' for doctors being trained in a new operation or procedure. It may take fifty procedures to perfect it, and if you are one of the patients in that first fifty, your chances of having a complication can be higher. The trouble is, we often don't know where our doctor is sitting on that learning curve. Asking 'How often have you done this operation or procedure?' is highly recommended.[12]

Despite there being no good quality evidence to support bone cement injections, the procedure has been approved by Australian health authorities to receive interim public funding under Medicare. Professor Rachelle Buchbinder feels that this approval will encourage 'easy access to an unproven treatment' and believes it should not be made widely available until it's proven. Part of the reason for the approval was because Dr Bill Clark was a member of the committee which recommended approval.[13] (Despite requests from one of the authors, Bill Clark declined to be quoted for this book.)

The committee in question is the Medical Services Advisory Committee, which looks at scientific evidence and recommends whether or not an operation or procedure warrants inclusion into Medicare, and thus receives public funding. It's similar to the Pharmaceutical Benefits Advisory Committee, which makes recommendations about whether a new drug should be included on the Pharmaceutical Benefits Scheme and made available to all Australians at a price they can afford. But as the case of vertebroplasty shows, procedures are not held to the same standards as pharmaceuticals. With no randomised controlled trials of injecting bone cement, it remains unproven and therefore potentially harmful to some people, and yet it is approved and available—albeit in a temporary way—under Medicare.

In reality, many new surgical procedures have not been tested in randomised controlled trials. In fact, if doctors were only allowed to do things that had been proven in such trials, a lot of things being done today would not be able to be continued. For example, in the fast-changing and high-tech world of interventional radiology, new techniques come and go quickly so it's very difficult to evaulate them in a high-quality way. In other words, there is no time to do rigorous long-term studies of new treatments and find out the long-term benefits and harms. The trouble is that many patients may have no idea that those rigorous studies haven't been undertaken. Ironically, once a procedure is widely used, it can be hard to conduct a randomised controlled trial. In the case of this procedure, doctors are finding it very hard to recruit trial participants.[14]

The tension between those who tend to promote this procedure and those pushing hard for rigorous evaluation highlights a much wider tension in medicine. Out there on the frontiers, doctors are doing all kinds of things that have not been proven in top-quality randomised controlled trials. To some people, they are visionaries and pioneers saving the lives and reducing the suffering of their patients. In the opinion of others, they are doing unproven things and may be risking patient safety. Medical pioneers take a lot of the public limelight, often deservedly so. But in recent decades, a new kind of doctor like Rachelle Buchbinder has been emerging. Influenced by a reform movement called 'evidence-based medicine', these doctors are passionately committed to treating patients, but they are also committed to evaluating those treatments. They want to be sure of the impact of treatments on patients, in both the short and long term. Arguments between these two camps have been raging inside the pages of medical journals for decades—mostly in polite and respectable tones. While it might seem to be an obscure debate between doctors, finding out more about 'evidence-based medicine' could be very good for your health. Asking questions like the ones featured in this book is one way to start joining in the conversation.

EXAMPLE 3
Caesarean or vaginal birth?

In many countries, more than 20 per cent of women are now giving birth by caesarean section. In Australia that means more than 50 000 women every year, with half of those caesareans being

Decision-aids can help weigh up harms and benefits

elective rather than happening due to an emergency.[15] In the United Kingdom the rates have doubled in nearly thirty years, from around 10 per cent in 1980 to more than 20 per cent today.[16] In the United States the figure is close to 30 per cent.[17] Rapidly rising rates of caesarean births mean more and more women are having to choose what they do with their subsequent births, and several decision aids have been developed to help women make those choices. The decisions the second time round can be extremely complicated, as either option—vaginal birth or caesarean—can harm the mother and baby. According to researchers who have looked closely at the evidence, vaginal birth is less risky—and also believed to be much less costly for the health system as a whole. But there is a strong view that women should be fully informed about the potential harms and benefits of either option, to enable them to make the decision that is best for them.

In the early 2000s, a group of Australian researchers developed a decision aid for pregnant women who had already had a caesarean delivery the first time round. The researchers summarised the best available evidence about the benefits and harms of both options and put it in plain language. The benefits of vaginal birth included: the overwhelming majority (up to 80 per cent) of attempted vaginal births did in fact succeed; the average length of stay in hospital was half of that for those having a caesarean; mother and baby avoided the risks of surgery; and vaginal birth led to a greater chance of successfully starting breastfeeding. The possible harms of vaginal birth included: an estimated 1 in 200 risk that already-existing tissue scar on the uterus would tear, causing potentially serious problems for mother and baby; the baby may need to be helped out by forceps; and many women may have a cut made in the lower part of the vagina to assist with the birth.[18]

For the caesarean option second time round, the benefits included: knowing what to expect; being able to plan in advance; and the fact that elective caesarean has lower rates of surgical complications, compared to an emergency caesarean. The risks of electing to have a caesarean included:

surgery associated pain; bleeding; infection of the wound or bladder; blood loss and blood clots; a longer stay in hospital; and a doubling of the risk of the baby experiencing short-term breathing problems from about 3 to 6 per cent.

In a small pilot study, the Australian researchers looking at the impact of using the decision aid found that most women felt it had helped them in making a choice. However, the study was too small to get a handle on how the decision aid would affect women more generally. A larger study followed.

In Britain, a study of more than 700 pregnant women using a similar decision aid found that it gave women greater knowledge and reduced their anxiety about making their choice.[19] It also tentatively found that after using one particular version of the decision aid, more women opted for vaginal birth. While the finding was tentative, the researchers concluded that if these aids were widely used by pregnant women who had already had a caesarean birth, it could mean 4000 fewer caesareans every year in England and Wales. It is possible that widespread use of these decision aids could help people get answers to their questions about harms and benefits at the same time as bringing an enormous cost saving to the health system.

Conclusion
Will this operation really help?

One of the big names of Australian medicine, Professor Stephen Leeder, from the University of Sydney, once dryly described surgery as a 'data-free zone'.[20] That was back in the

1990s but, as the examples in this chapter highlight, there are still commonly used operations and procedures that have not been properly tested, so there is no good scientific data to help people make decisions. The argument from many of the surgeons who undertake these procedures is that it would be unethical to conduct a randomised controlled trial because that would mean denying half the people in the trial the potentially beneficial operation. It's a powerful argument which may sound convincing. But without good trials, our choices will be more like stabbing in the dark than making fully informed decisions in the light of good evidence. If an operation or procedure is unproven, it doesn't mean it is useless or harmful, it just means it's unproven. It is, however, important that patients know how thoroughly treatments have been tested, and whether they are undergoing a well-proven operation or a risky experimental procedure.

Many of us find it difficult to ask tough questions of experienced and confident surgeons. But if your life or that of your loved one depends on it, it may well be worth making the effort. Besides, these days it's fair enough to expect surgeons, like other health professionals, to be prepared to answer such questions. It is part and parcel of good practice.

More questions about operations

Will this operation (or procedure) really help?

- What are the risks and benefits?
- What happens if I do nothing?
- What other options are there?
- What can I do beforehand to prepare myself for this procedure?
- What can I do afterwards to maximise my chances of recovery?
- How well has this operation or procedure been tested?
- Have there been many randomised controlled trials?
- Is there a systematic review of the evidence available?
- How often have you done this operation or procedure?
- What back-up is available at this hospital or unit if things go wrong?
- Is there a decision aid available about this operation or procedure?

SOME GENERAL
QUESTIONS TO
CONSIDER

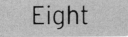

Eight

What is the evidence?

Many treatments and tests in widespread use are not backed by strong evidence that they do more good than harm. Asking the simple question 'What is the evidence that this treatment or test will help me?' may save you from having unnecessary, costly or even harmful treatments and tests. It is worth developing a basic understanding of the different types of studies used in health and medical research. This understanding of the different types of evidence will help you to be more informed when making health decisions. When the health and medical industry, the media or other groups are promoting tests and treatments, this knowledge will also help you to ask questions that may be life-saving.

It's no wonder if you sometimes feel confused about what is good for your health and what is not. It seems as though every day brings another news story about some medical discovery that contradicts yesterday's discovery. One day, we are warned against eating too much red meat. The next day, another scientist is urging us to eat more meat. One day, we are told of an exciting breakthrough in the quest to prevent heart disease. And then we hear that this so-called revolutionary treatment has turned out to be more harmful than helpful. One doctor suggests that you take a particular medicine, but another warns against it. How can we make sense of this overwhelming tide of conflicting and contradictory statements about our health, and of what treatments we should, or should not, be trying?

The answer is simpler than you might think. And the good news is that you don't have to be a scientist, a doctor or a professor to make sense of health information. All you need is a basic understanding of the different types of studies used in scientific and health research. This will help you to assess the reliability of much health advice, whether it is coming from the television news, your neighbour or your doctor. It will also equip you to ask important questions of doctors or anyone else suggesting you try a particular test, treatment or therapy. Asking questions—such as, 'What is the evidence for this recommendation?'—may save you from having unnecessary, costly or even harmful treatments, or help ensure that you don't miss out on therapies which may make an important difference to your life.

Broadly speaking, you can divide health and medical research into four broad categories:

(1) laboratory studies;
(2) observational studies;

(3) randomised controlled trials; and

(4) systematic reviews or meta-analyses.

It is well worth trying to become a little more familiar with these different sorts of studies, and discussing them with your doctor or other health professional.

The first category includes laboratory-based studies—those involving experiments on animals or human tissue or cells, for example. These are extremely important for **Be sceptical about medical promotion** providing insights into the causes of diseases and identifying potential treatments. But it can be a mistake to assume that because something has been shown to have a positive impact in a test tube or in animal experiments that this means it will also apply to humans. The old saying about cancer—that it has been cured countless times in rodents—is a reminder that what works in other species will not necessarily work for humans. Yet we so often hear media reports of 'scientific breakthroughs' which inspire great hope in patients and their families. Unfortunately, an important development in scientific knowledge does not necessarily translate into an important development for patients.

Often these stories are driven by vested interests—companies or others that stand to gain from promoting encouraging findings about their products or services. And when you dig deeper into these reports, you often discover that they are based on very early findings, the implications of which are far from clear. They may be describing laboratory results, so what they might mean for your health—or anyone else's—is usually uncertain.

One recent analysis—comparing the results of studies conducted on animals and humans for six different treatments—found that in half of the cases, the animal studies reached different conclusions to the human studies.[1] For example, animal studies suggested that treating head injuries with drugs called corticosteroids would be beneficial. But treating people on the basis of these successful animal experiments would have led to unnecessary deaths. The analysis also found that many animal studies are poorly designed and conducted, meaning that their results may not be reliable even when the animals being studied are useful models for disease in humans.

But this doesn't stop the media from reporting the findings of preliminary or poor quality studies as 'breakthrough'. Reports about breakthroughs help sell newspapers and boost television and radio ratings. There is widespread concern that overly promotional media reporting of research and treatments not only arouses false hope amongst patients but also encourages the use of harmful or ineffective treatments. The news is not all bad, however. As we shall see in the first example, a number of projects around the world are working to encourage better reporting of health and medical research. These projects are asking the tough questions about media reports that you can also be asking when you hear stories in the news on medical developments. They can help you make sense of the question, 'What is the evidence?'

The second broad category of health and medical research covers what are called 'observational studies'. These are studies examining differences between groups of people. Researchers may follow different groups of people over a period of time and examine relationships between their health and what they eat, how they behave or what medicines they take. Or they may just look at the differences between groups of people at a particular point in time—for example, whether people being admitted to hospital for heart surgery are smokers or not. These types of studies can provide useful information and hints about the causes and cures of many health problems. But they generally cannot provide high-level proof of cause and effect. They can't prove that taking a certain pill or eating red meat or living on a highway will, for example, have any predictable impact on health. In other words, it can be a mistake to conclude that you will live longer if you take vitamins just because observational studies have found people who take vitamins tend to live longer than people who do not. It is possible that other factors explain their long lives. It may be, for example, that people who take vitamins tend to also be more physically active or wealthier than people who do not, and these other factors may account for their longer lives.

This brings us to the third broad category of studies, which provide more reliable evidence about the impact of treatments. They are known as randomised controlled trials or RCTs because they randomly allocate people to different types of treatment and/or a placebo (an inactive or dummy treatment). Because people have been randomly allocated to different groups at the start of the study, this helps ensure that any differences observed between the groups at the end of the study are due to the differences in their treatment, rather than other factors.

Ideally, both the researchers and the people who are participating in these trials do not know until the end of the trial which group is having which treatment. This aims to overcome a natural human bias to which we are all vulnerable. Whether we are researchers conducting a study or patients taking part in a study, there is a natural tendency to believe in the power of a treatment. This is called the placebo effect. It is why many randomised controlled trials give one of the groups a placebo—so as to measure the impact of a treatment above and beyond any placebo effect.

In recent years, researchers and doctors have become more aware of the importance of conducting proper randomised controlled trials of treatments. While many doctors once were happy to recommend the use of treatments such as hormone replacement therapy on the basis of observational studies, it is now widely recognised that this approach led to a large number of women paying an extremely high price. Thousands of women around the world suffered cancers, heart attacks and strokes as a result of this premature enthusiasm for hormone replacement therapy. As shown in the second example, peoples' lives can be jeopardised by the use of treatments which are not backed by good quality evidence from randomised controlled trials. If more women had known to ask a simple question of their doctors—'Has this hormone replacement therapy been proven to be safe and effective in large randomised controlled trials?'—then perhaps much suffering and many deaths could have been prevented.

The fourth broad category of research includes studies known as systematic reviews. This means that the results of all studies on a known topic, which meet certain criteria about their quality, are summarised. Systematic reviews generally provide more reliable information than any single study, so you can generally be more confident about health advice based on a meta-analysis or a systematic review than if it is based on a single study. But systematic reviews can include many different types of studies, including basic scientific research, observational studies and randomised controlled trials. As you've probably gathered by now, a systematic review including randomised controlled trials will generally be more reliable than one based on observational studies.

At first glance, all of this information about the different types of studies can sound overwhelming. But it's worth taking a bit of time to get your head around it. Just knowing a few simple questions to ask when a treatment is recommended—such as, 'what sort of evidence is available to show this treatment is helpful and safe?'—can make all the difference. If the answer is 'good-quality randomised controlled trials', you can be more confident about the merits of the treatment. Of course, how you weigh up the benefits and harms of any treatment will depend on your individual situation. If you are battling a serious illness, you may be more willing to risk a treatment that has not yet been properly tested, and may cause harm. But if your problem is not so critical, you may be less willing to chance suffering serious side effects.

It is also worth remembering that knowledge is not static. What seems certain today may seem less certain tomorrow, when the results of further research become available. It is worth keeping in mind that knowledge is rarely set in concrete, but is likely to evolve and develop over time.

Be cautious about other peoples' stories

Sometimes when you're sick or having to make decisions about a treatment, it can seem as though everyone you know has advice to offer. Friends, neighbours, acquaintances and colleagues will often suggest you try a treatment because it worked for them or someone they know. This type of information is known as anecdotal evidence. It can be very persuasive: someone's story about their experience with an illness or treatment will often sound more convincing than the statistical findings of large studies involving people you've never met.

But anecdotal evidence based on the stories of individuals can be dangerously misleading. While systematic reviews based on randomised controlled trials provide the most reliable forms of evidence, anecdotal evidence is generally the least reliable. Just because a treatment seems to have worked for one person does not mean that it really did. And, even if it did work for one person, this does not mean it will work for you. If someone got better after taking a particular treatment, you can't always be sure that it was that treatment which really made a difference. Perhaps they would have recovered anyway, or maybe it was something else they did that was responsible for their improvement. There's also another issue: if someone tells you that their cancer was cured because they took a certain treatment, you may not be hearing from the nine other people who also took the treatment but didn't survive.

Yet personal testimony is often used to promote health products, particularly in the field of complementary or alternative medicines. Traditionally, mainstream science has neglected complementary health treatments, and we haven't had reliable evidence to show whether these treatments are helpful or harmful. Luckily, more and more research is now examining these treatments. Sometimes they are not as effective as their promoters would have you believe. One example of this comes from the widespread use of saw palmetto for prostate disease, as discussed in the third example. It's important to ask the question 'What is the evidence?', whether someone is suggesting you have surgery, take a prescription medicine or try an alternative health product.

EXAMPLE 1
Media warning

The media went wild when news broke in the late 1990s that scientists were developing a new treatment for the common cold. The experimental drug was widely described by journalists as a cure, a miracle, a magic bullet, a wonder drug, a super drug and a medical first. It was compared with the search for the Holy Grail and man's landing on the moon. In the United States alone, around 1000 newspaper articles and television reports trumpeted the 'breakthrough' news about the drug, called pleconaril, between 1997 and 2002.[2] Most reports didn't mention or were dismissive of any potential for side effects.

Headlines can be misleading

Not surprisingly, all this positive publicity was very healthy for the stock price of ViroPharma Inc., the company developing pleconaril. There was just one little hitch. The company's application to market the drug in the United States was rejected in 2002. Not only did randomised controlled trials show that the drug was not very effective, it had the potential to cause serious side effects. The company abandoned its work on pleconaril soon afterwards. But these setbacks didn't attract nearly so much media interest— headlines about 'Cold Drug No Breakthrough' are not nearly as enticing to newspaper editors or their audiences as those promising 'Breakthrough Cures Cold'.

It may seem amazing that so many journalists and media outlets could have been gullible enough to promote a product as a miracle cure before its scientific merits were even known. But unfortunately, this is not an isolated case. The media is often guilty of acting like a marketing arm of the pharmaceutical, medical and complementary health industries. Many media outlets have shown themselves ready and willing to report something as true just because it is said by a doctor, scientist or other health professional. They often fail to ask the hard question: 'What is the evidence for your claim?'

Journalists also often fail to tell their audiences that they are covering a story because of a public relations or marketing campaign by a vested interest, such as a company seeking to promote its product or a hospital seeking to promote its services. Investigations by the United States–based non-profit organisation Center for Media and Democracy have found that the television news sometimes runs video reports produced by public relations firms for corporate clients as if they are news.[3]

The media can also mislead its audiences by failing to distinguish between the different types of studies: reports based on preliminary findings from animal studies can be given as much weight and prominence on a TV news bulletin as those based on more reliable findings from large randomised controlled trials. When journalists and editors are deciding which stories to cover or to feature prominently, they often fail to consider whether the story is based on good evidence from a reliable study. They are usually more interested in running a story that is likely to interest and attract audiences than in choosing a story because it is based on reliable evidence.

Many experts are concerned that overly promotional media reporting is encouraging people to try treatments and tests whose benefits may be uncertain or whose use may be unnecessary or even harmful. Sharing such concerns is a United States journalist with long-standing experience in covering health issues, Gary Schwitzer, Assistant Professor at the University of Minnesota School of Journalism and Mass Communication. Schwitzer believes that words like 'cure' and 'breakthrough' should be banned from media reports about health and medicine.[4] 'When journalists write about cures, it's difficult to be sure what is meant,' he says. 'Does it mean absence of disease? Does it mean no recurrence of once-existing disease? Does it mean today, next week, five years, or a "normal life expectancy"?' Similarly, Schwitzer says it's difficult to know what is meant when journalists (or doctors and scientists) call something a 'breakthrough'. It can take years before it's known whether something described as a breakthrough really is one. Too often, new treatments described as breakthroughs turn out to do less good and more harm than was initially expected.

If you see or hear terms like these being used in a media report about some new development in research or treatments, it pays to be wary. Don't take the story on face value, and certainly don't make any health decisions based on what you hear from the media. These days, with the Internet and the ready availability of global knowledge, it doesn't take too much effort to check out the reliability of media reports and the quality of evidence upon which they are based. When you read media reports, some helpful questions to consider include: 'Has this study been published in a reputable journal?' and 'Who is promoting this study, and why?' You might also ask: 'Why is the media covering this story? Is it because someone is trying to sell me something?' and 'Does this media report talk about the potential harms as well as potential benefits of the treatment or test?'

In fact, several projects around the world now provide objective, up-to-date, online assessment of media reporting of health news. If you are interested in finding out more about the evidence behind a treatment or test that's been reported in the news, it's worth having a look at such websites in case they've already examined the issue.

For assessments of media reporting of health news, look at:

- **Media Doctor Australia: <www.mediadoctor.org.au>**
- **Media Doctor Canada: <www.mediadoctor.ca>**
- **Hitting the Headlines, UK: <www.library.nhs.uk>**
- **Health News Review (United States): <www.HealthNewsReview.org>**

These sites also give a good general introduction to the sorts of questions you should ask about media reports to help assess their reliability. Being sceptical about what you read or hear from the media might save you from having unnecessary, costly or even harmful tests or treatments.

EXAMPLE 2
Hormone replacement therapy

For decades, millions of women around the world were encouraged to take hormone replacement therapy (HRT) for years at a time. They were told this would reduce their risk of heart attack, stroke and other problems that can develop after the menopause.

When concerns were raised that it may also increase their chance of getting breast cancer, these were often dismissed on the grounds that this risk was worth taking because the potential benefits—in reducing heart disease—were so much greater.

Misleading evidence has been used to promote harmful drugs to women

We now know that many women paid a high price for the medical industry's overenthusiastic promotion of HRT. It turned out that long-term use of HRT, rather than preventing heart attacks and strokes, increased the risk of these often lethal conditions, while also increasing breast cancer risk.

These days, there is widespread agreement that HRT should only be used in the lowest possible dose for the shortest time needed to relieve menopause symptoms. In other words, it should be used only for short-term relief of symptoms associated with menopause rather than as a long-term preventative of heart disease.

The HRT saga raises many awkward questions for modern medicine, including: How could drugs which were so widely prescribed to otherwise healthy women (HRT was promoted for preventing disease, remember) turn out to be harmful? At least part of the answer lies in understanding the different types of evidence used to back the use of HRT over the years.

Suggestions that HRT might reduce the risk of heart disease and osteoporosis came from laboratory research and studies looking at the medication's effect on blood components and bone thickness. But these studies were not capable of answering more important questions such as whether taking HRT long term would stop people from suffering from these diseases or dying from them. Although the early studies were promising, they were not proof of benefit. As we've discussed, there are plenty of examples from other areas of medicine where treatments that look promising in early studies are later shown in more rigorous studies to have no benefit or even to do harm.

Studies observing the differences between women who elected to take HRT and those who didn't were also promising. But as with the laboratory studies mentioned above, these observational studies did not prove the benefits of HRT. Women who chose to take HRT were also healthier in other ways, and these types of studies were not capable of proving it was the HRT which was responsible for their better health.

What was missing during the decades when long-term HRT use was being promoted was evidence from randomised controlled trials to assess its benefits and safety. This lack of evidence did not, however, stop the pharmaceutical industry from vigorously marketing their lucrative products. Many of the doctors promoting widespread HRT use were probably well-intentioned, and familiar with its benefits in relieving distressing menopausal symptoms. But undoubtedly, some were also influenced, even if subconsciously, by their ties with industry.

When a visiting US expert told an Australian newspaper in the early 1990s that all women over fifty should be on long-term HRT for protection against heart disease and osteoporosis, his was not a lone voice. Some medical organisations were making similar recommendations, and an article in a respected Australian medical journal said it was appropriate for doctors 'to discuss the option of HRT with most menopausal women'.[5] Similarly, the American Medical Association published a consumer book in 1998, *The Essential Guide to Menopause*, saying that most doctors believed HRT was beneficial for most women. In Australia, the National Health and Medical Research Council said in a 1996 media statement that 'the potential benefits from the treatment in preventing coronary heart disease and osteoporosis more than offset any possible small increase in the risk of breast cancer'.

With such widespread promotion of HRT, it is not surprising that, by 2002, more than 60 million women in the US alone were taking the two top-selling brands.

Ironically, when proposals were first floated to run a large randomised controlled trial to properly evaluate the impact of HRT—the now famous Women's Health Initiative study—some doctors argued it was unethical to give women a placebo when hormones were so beneficial.

When the study began, most concerns about HRT were centred on worries it increased the risk of breast cancer. The first significant doubts about its role in preventing heart disease arose with a systematic review published in 1997, showing that HRT did not reduce heart attacks in women with established heart disease and may even increase them.[6] These results were such a shock that many doctors had difficulty believing them, instead emphasising that they were applicable only to women with established heart disease and there was no reason to stop using HRT to prevent heart disease in healthy women.

In 2002, the medical and menopause industry was stunned when the Women's Health Initiative study, the first randomised controlled trial to evaluate HRT in preventing disease in healthy women, was stopped three years earlier than planned because early results suggested the therapy was doing more harm than good. Any potential benefits were outweighed by an increased incidence of heart disease, stroke, blood clots, gallbladder disease, incontinence, dementia and breast cancer.[7] The findings triggered a massive controversy. Many doctors who had built their careers on the back of the menopause industry found it difficult to accept the results.

For many women and their families, the medical industry's premature enthusiasm for HRT resulted in unnecessary deaths and suffering. It may not be a coincidence that breast cancer diagnoses dropped in many countries after publicity about the Women's Health Initiative study prompted tens of millions of women to abandon HRT.[8]

The HRT story is a reminder that a misplaced belief in the power of pills can divert attention from other ways of improving health. When doctors are busy prescribing pills for menopause, they have less time to recommend different options for relieving such symptoms, such as exercise, lifestyle changes, or even reassuring patients that most menopause symptoms will eventually disappear of their own accord.

The HRT tragedy is also a sobering reminder of the importance of being sceptical when treatments are being promoted, even if it is by a respected professor. The National Women's Health Network in the US, which helped push for proper evaluation of HRT, says its rise and fall has sweeping implications for medicine, and that 'pharmaceutical interventions should not be inflicted on healthy people until these interventions are proven safe and effective in randomized controlled trials'.[9]

The other lesson is that we cannot always rely on our doctors or the medical establishment to ask the tough questions on our behalf. You need to know what questions to ask, including: 'Are there any systematic reviews of randomised controlled trials or decision aids that spell out the potential benefits and harms of this treatment?'

EXAMPLE 3
Benign prostate disease

Asking about evidence is also important for complementary therapies

Stories like the hormone replacement therapy saga have contributed to a growing public scepticism about modern medicine and its ties to the pharmaceutical industry. This mistrust has encouraged many people to turn to the alternative or complementary health sector.

As well, many people are drawn by the promise that 'natural' products are gentler and thus less likely to cause side effects. But it can be a mistake to put your faith in such promises. Alternative and complementary health products and practices can be harmful. After all, if a product is powerful enough to have a therapeutic effect, it may also cause side effects.

People often say they prefer natural health products 'because they don't contain chemicals'. But of course they do. And the substances found in plants and nature can be just as toxic as those made by humans. After all, one of a plant's major defence mechanisms against predators is to try to poison them. There are many examples of natural health products causing harm, whether because of a reaction to the product itself or because the product is not what it claims to be. Studies of natural health products and medicines have found undeclared pharmaceuticals or contaminants such as lead, mercury and arsenic.

Some complementary medicine experts argue that traditional remedies, such as Chinese herbal medicine, have withstood the test of time and so must be safe. Far fewer adverse reactions are reported for complementary than prescription medicines, but this may reflect, at least partly, that reporting of such problems was not formally encouraged until recently. As well, rare but serious complications have emerged in herbs which have been used for thousands of years and previously been considered safe. Modern production methods may differ from traditional methods, while many manufacturers are combining herbs that were not used together traditionally. As well, the effects of traditional medicines may vary between populations who have used them for centuries and those which have different genetic make-ups and dietary habits.

In other words, being sceptical about the claims made by those promoting complementary health products and services may save more than just your wallet. It may also save you from nasty side effects. The complementary health sector is a billion-dollar industry, which includes companies just as dedicated to promoting their wares as any other profit-driven business. When the pharmaceutical industry funds research, that research is likely to provide the results that the industry wants for its marketing and sales. And the same is true for research funded by the complementary health industry.

Many of the questions that you should ask about mainstream medical treatments are also relevant for complementary treatments. Once it might have been difficult to have such questions answered, as scientific and medical research traditionally neglected the complementary sector. However, growing awareness of the popularity of these treatments is encouraging more rigorous evaluation of them. Now, you only have to switch on your computer to track down high-quality studies about the impact of such common treatments as acupuncture and herbal products. (See the recommended reading list at the end of this book for some websites.)

Sometimes, the results of these studies may come as a surprise—especially if you are one of the many men who has been shelling out your hard-earned dollars on a popular herbal treatment for a prostate problem common in older men. The treatment is based on extracts from the fruit of saw palmetto, a slow-growing, long-living palm that goes by the scientific name of *Serenoa repens*. Widely promoted as a treatment for benign prostate hyperplasia, an extremely annoying condition in which swelling of the prostate causes difficulties with urine flow, it is not surprising that men have been very receptive to promises made by the dozens of websites selling saw palmetto. In the United States alone, it is estimated that more than 2 million men regularly take such products.

What many of the websites promoting saw palmetto fail to mention is an important trial published in 2006 in the *New England Journal of Medicine*.[10] In this study, 225 men over the age of 49 with moderate to severe prostate problems were randomly allocated to take either saw palmetto extract (160 mg twice daily) or a placebo pill for one year. At the end of the year, there was no significant difference between the two groups of men, suggesting that saw palmetto was no more effective than a placebo. The researchers noted that previous studies had suggested some benefit from the product, but said many of these studies had been small, lasted only short periods of time or were poorly designed. On the other hand, it is possible that because the later study used one specific saw palmetto product, its results may not be relevant for other preparations.

This study does not provide the final answer to questions about the usefulness or otherwise of saw palmetto. Single studies rarely provide definitive answers; these usually come only when enough well-conducted studies have been completed, reviewed and summarised in a systematic review. But it certainly raises a question about the merits of a widely used treatment. It also shows the importance of not taking promotional claims at face value. A cursory search of the Internet would have revealed the results of this study, even if they were not mentioned in many of the product advertisements.

It is a reminder that no matter who is promoting a treatment, and no matter what the type of treatment being recommended, it is worth taking the time and effort to ask questions about the quality of evidence to back the claims being made. One important question to ask is: 'What is the evidence to support the treatment or test that is being recommended?'

Conclusion

What is the evidence?

Many men may still decide to try saw palmetto even if they are aware of the uncertainties surrounding its effects on prostate symptoms. The point of this chapter is not to argue that you should agree only to have treatments or tests that are backed by high-quality evidence showing they are safe and effective. The reality is that in far more cases than you might expect, this evidence is not available because the proper studies have not been done. In these situations, you will have to weigh up the uncertainties involved.

Even if the evidence is conclusive in suggesting that a treatment is unlikely to have major benefits, you may still decide it is worth taking the chance that it will help. But it is far better to make this decision on the basis of the best available evidence. And no matter how convincing the evidence to support the use of a test or treatment, this is no guarantee of how it will work for you. All that we can learn from even the best quality studies is the probability that a treatment will have a certain effect. If good-quality studies show that seven out of ten people benefit from taking a particular treatment, there is no guarantee that it will work for you. You may be one of the 30 per cent who are not helped.

Developing a basic understanding of the different types of scientific evidence will help you to start asking some vital questions. If you find it difficult to ask these questions of your doctor or other health professionals, the Internet has opened up a whole new world for patients and their families. You now have access to information that was once the exclusive domain of doctors and researchers. Knowing a bit about the reliability of different types of studies will help you to find your way around this brave new world, and to ask the sorts of questions that could make all the difference to your health and well-being. Don't fall for the hype, whatever the type of treatment or test being promoted.

More questions about the evidence

What is the evidence?

- Has this study been published in a reputable journal?
- Who funded this study?
- Who is promoting this study, and why?
- How reliable is this health information?
- Is it being pushed by a vested interest?
- Are there any systematic reviews of randomised controlled trials or decision aids that spell out the potential benefits and harms of this treatment?
- Why is the media covering this story? Is it because someone is trying to sell me something?
- Does this media report talk about the potential harms as well as potential benefits of the treatment or test?
- What is the evidence to support the treatment or test that is being recommended?

Nine

Who else is profiting here?

Sadly, health care is often driven by the profit motive. Too many doctors are taking money and other gifts from drug companies seeking to maximise drug sales, and this can influence what drugs they prescribe for you. Increasingly, influential patient groups are also on the gravy train, helping promote new treatments and keeping a little too quiet when their sponsors' products turn out not to be the miracle cures they were marketed to be. Meanwhile, some doctors working for private medical corporations are recommending tests and procedures to help improve the corporate bottom line, rather than your health. Asking 'Who else is profiting here?' can produce some alarming answers.

Try to imagine a world where slick sales reps from drug companies take senior specialists out on the town, spend hundreds of dollars on them, and end up at lap-dancing joints late at night. Then try to imagine a time when most patient groups around the world are funded by pharmaceutical companies. And now imagine a giant private hospital corporation getting so greedy that one of its leading surgeons starts performing costly surgery on people who don't need it. As you've probably already guessed, there's no need to imagine, because these tales are all true. This sort of corruption is endemic within the world of medicine and science. Behind the scenes there are massive financial forces at work, trying to influence your doctor to prescribe you the latest most expensive pill, or send you for a costly and potentially dangerous procedure, when you may be better off doing nothing. Whenever someone suggests you need a test, a pill or an operation, it is often worth asking: 'Who else is profiting here?'

Pharmaceutical industry marketing strategies now influence and distort virtually every aspect of medical life, drug and device companies fund a majority of patient groups, and private for-profit medical companies are constantly being caught out either denying people the care they need or giving too much care to those who don't need it. Asking questions about the financial dealings of your doctor, patient support group or medical centre may seem like a big ask, but the answers revealed could shock you.

For several years now, the world's leading medical journals have been publishing article after article highlighting the dangers of doctors being too cosy with drug companies. Almost every researcher who looks into this issue finds that when doctors accept 'food, flattery and friendship' from drug companies, those doctors' decisions become fundamentally distorted.[1] While many drug company products can save lives, some of their marketing strategies can be poisonous. Drunk under the influence of marketing, doctors may prescribe an expensive new drug when another remedy might be far better, safer and cheaper. No one who looks at this issue dispassionately can seriously question these findings any more: the debate has now moved on to how to stop the seduction and put an end to the wining and dining. But until the money and the wine stops flowing, the only way you will find out if your doctor is still on the gravy train will be to ask them directly: 'What are your links with drug companies?'

A few years ago the *British Medical Journal* ran an entire issue on the subject, with the plain-talking title: 'Time to untangle doctors from drug companies'.[2] More recently, across the other side of the Atlantic, the *Journal of the American Medical Association* carried a watershed article calling for a major clean-up and an end to most of the corrupting financial ties.[3] At the same time, the *Medical Journal of Australia* published a piece called 'Doctors behaving badly?', which argued that doctors should be completely up-front with their patients about every single gift they receive.[4]

The point of asking your doctor about all of his or her gifts, trips away, expensive restaurant experiences and attendance at sponsored education is not to embarrass or shame them. The point is that doctors who accept these sorts of gifts do not tend to give you the best care, and you or your loved ones may want to know that before you sit down to a consultation. Despite the inevitable claim that 'I can take the money and maintain my independence', there is a mountain of good scientific evidence showing that accepting the gifts in fact distorts doctors' decisions and it makes them more likely to prescribe the drug made by the gift-giver.[5] It's common sense: why would drug companies bother to splash out on all those lavish meals if it wasn't going to pay off in extra sales? And while drug companies get a lot of attention, as we will see in the first example, the companies making medical devices and high-tech equipment are also very good at trying to seduce surgeons into using their products.

Increasingly, patient groups and medical foundations are playing a bigger role in the health system. These groups can raise money for research, write important reports, lobby governments, produce information for the public, and speak to the media about the latest treatments. But it's often not clear that groups raising awareness about a particular disease usually accept money from the companies who make drugs for that disease. It makes perfect sense but, as the second example shows, it can lead to unhealthy conflicts of interest. One problem is that, even in a well-meaning way, patient groups can tend towards exaggeration of how widespread or serious a particular condition is, and can also overplay the benefits of its sponsors' drug. Perhaps worst of all, patient groups or medical foundations can sometimes seem to temporarily lose their voice when their sponsors' drugs are found to have serious side effects. If you are thinking of getting involved with a group or even just relying on their information, it is well worth asking about their links with companies or other vested interests.

One of the age-old problems within health care is that healers tend to profit from doing *something* rather than *nothing*, particularly in countries like the United States where the private sector plays a big role. A surgeon working in private practice will make money every time they recommend surgery to their patients—the more operations, the bigger their profits. A naturopath who sells herbs out of their clinic makes money every time they prescribe herbs—the more herbs they prescribe, the bigger their profits. Doctors who own giant testing machines make money every time you are sent for a test—the more tests, the

Private medical centres and hospital corporations can profit from unnecessary tests and treatments

bigger the profits. This doesn't mean we should never trust our health professionals, it just means it's worth thinking about who else is profiting from treating our illnesses. Making this age-old problem far worse is the rise and rise of giant private medical corporations, which develop very sophisticated methods of maximising profits. As we will see in the third example, it could be profitable for you to ask about the ownership of medical centres and hospitals where you receive treatment.

EXAMPLE 1
Doctors and drug companies

Don't believe anyone who tells you that the days of drug companies wining and dining doctors are over. Not so long ago, a couple of employees from the giant American drug company Abbott were taking a hospital specialist to a lap-dancing club in Britain.[6] Around the same time, Swiss drug giant Roche was footing the bill for a $200-a-head dinner for hundreds of cancer doctors at one of Australia's fanciest restaurants, at the Sydney Opera House.[7] Meanwhile, in the United States, one of the biggest medical device manufacturers was allegedly spending millions of dollars annually on bribes and other perks for spine surgeons.[8]

Too many doctors are drunk on drug company money

If you get a group of doctors talking informally, and if they think they won't be quoted, most of them can tell stories about the attempts at seduction by vested interests so extreme that you simply wouldn't believe them. From the beginning as medical students, much of their drinking and dining is funded directly by companies who stand to profit from what those doctors will recommend to you, their patients. And it's much, much more than expensive dinners and good wine. When they are out of medical school and into practice, doctors are bombarded by visits from friendly sales reps every week. Then they undertake so-called 'continuing medical education'— often accompanied by lavish meals—courtesy of the drug companies. They attend 'scientific' seminars fully sponsored by drug and device manufacturers and are often flown around the country and the world all expenses-paid—with the tabs again picked up by the companies marketing the latest high-tech product or pill. In Australia, drug companies sponsor perhaps 30 000 such events a year. In the United States, the figure is more than 300 000.

While enormous attention is paid to the links between drug companies and doctors, the problem is of course much wider with the connections between surgeons and the makers of surgical devices receiving increasing attention. Similarly, the world of complementary medicine may be just as vulnerable to the influence of vested interests, with giant companies sponsoring scientific symposia on alternative remedies.[9]

Accepting a gift—whether it be a meal or a trip—naturally makes a human being want to return the favour. The best way for a doctor to return the favour to a drug company sales representative is to prescribe that company's products to as many patients as possible. If that latest expensive drug happens to be the best for their patients, then everybody is a winner. But it is often the case that there are better options available—including cheaper medicines or no treatment at all. With high blood pressure for example, existing cheaper drugs called thiazides have been shown to work just as well for many patients as the newer more expensive ones, but they are far less widely prescribed. In situations where health dollars are limited (and that's most of the world, really), using a new expensive drug when a cheaper one would do just as well can mean a death sentence for those who miss out on life-saving therapy because scarce resources have been squandered.

And what's becoming increasingly clear is that it's not just individual doctors who are influenced by all the gifts they receive: much of the scientific evidence itself has become fundamentally compromised because so many medical studies and clinical trials are now funded directly by drug companies. Research has shown that studies funded by a drug company or other vested interests are far more likely to yield a positive result than studies funded by more independent sources.[10] This has led some people to suggest there is a 'systematic bias' in the scientific literature that doctors use to base their decisions on. This bias means doctors have an overly optimistic view of how much a drug will help. As you start to use that scientific literature, it could be valuable to ask yourself: 'Who has funded this study?' Often you will find the answer in small print at the end of a journal article. Just because it is funded by a company does not mean it is necessarily biased or unreliable; however, drug company sponsorship does tend to mean that the results will paint the drug in a more favourable light—and will tend to exaggerate benefits and play down harms.

As more and more public scandals have erupted over doctors having their stethoscopes in the trough, medical journals have become tougher and tougher about ensuring that authors of scientific papers disclose their financial ties to drug companies and other vested interests. If you read journal articles regularly, you will find it is not uncommon for doctors to disclose that they have taken money from half a dozen drug companies or more. Those disclosures do not yet include how much money they receive, but sometimes it is a very large amount. New laws in a few states of the United States now require drug companies to disclose how much they pay doctors—and some have received up to US$1 million a year.[11]

But while doctors have to disclose their financial ties to medical journals before they publish an article, they do not have to routinely disclose it to their patients—who really have the biggest need to know. Two Australian researchers have recently proposed that doctors should disclose all gifts they receive from private companies, perhaps on a wall chart in their surgeries.[12] The plan includes naming both the individual companies doing the wining and dining, and the latest drugs that those companies are marketing. Doctors would have to write down every single lunch and dinner, every sponsored scientific seminar and every all-expenses-paid trip away. The idea makes a lot of sense as it would allow patients to see for the first time the full extent of drug company influence over their supposedly independent doctors.

Such full disclosure would also benefit the growing numbers of doctors who are cutting all their ties to drug companies. Many organisations around the world are suggesting that doctors stop seeing drug representatives and going to 'educational' dinners funded by drug companies. Groups like No Free Lunch and Healthy Skepticism have been arguing for more separation between doctors and drug companies for many years.[13] An article in the *Journal of the American Medical Association* in 2006 suggested that many of the current links between doctors and for-profit companies should be totally prohibited at medical centres attached to universities in the United States.[14]

Until doctors and other health professionals are required to disclose all their relevant financial ties—or, better, to end them—the best way for you to find out about them is simply to ask. This is, of course, not an easy task. Many people can be defensive about these sorts of relationships, and even asking the question can cause offence. However, the more often these questions are asked, the easier the asking will become. Good medical journalists now routinely try to question the doctors they interview about their links to drug companies, and then try to include that information in the stories they write.

Ultimately, though, we will probably need tough new laws making it illegal for doctors to accept gifts from those with a vested interest in what those doctors recommend to their patients. Judges can't accept fancy lunches from those whose claims they are evaluating, so why should doctors be able to?

EXAMPLE 2

Patient groups and drug companies

Many patient groups have conflicts of interest too

When the new 'wonder drugs' to treat arthritis hit the market a few years back, arthritis groups around the world celebrated. Often with sponsorship from the companies promoting new arthritis drugs, known as COX-2s, some of these patient groups and foundations helped run advertising campaigns and made excited statements in the media. A new era in the treatment of pain was apparently dawning. A few short years later, those same drugs were at the centre of a major international scandal (see chapter 6, 'What are the side effects?', for the full story).

As the truth about these drugs emerged, their benefits were shown to be far less dramatic than first claimed and their harms were, for some people, extremely serious. In at least one case, a drug was taken off the market because of concerns about its safety. Funnily enough, expressions of concern about these harms by patient groups—at least in Australia—did not appear to match the celebration accompanying the arrival of the new class of drugs a few years earlier. You don't bite the hand that feeds you.[15]

A recent global survey suggested perhaps two-thirds of patient support groups receive some funding from drug companies or device manufacturers.[16] Suggestions that the sponsorship comes without strings attached are as naive as they are absurd. There are many documented examples of patient groups and medical foundations becoming intertwined with the marketing campaigns of their generous sponsors. In 2006, the giant drug company GSK was found to have breached an industry code of practice in Britain after it used a patient support group's website to promote a drug for 'restless legs syndrome', even though the drug was not yet licensed.[17] The highly successful United States–based consumer advocacy group Children and Adults with Attention Deficit Hyperactivity Disorder (CHADD) began its life with large grants from the makers of Ritalin, and to this day still relies on the pharmaceutical industry for close to A$1 million a year.[18] The Swiss-based International Osteoporosis Foundation also heavily relies on partnerships with drug companies and has used celebrities to help sell messages that synchronise with the industry's marketing campaigns.[19]

In Australia, when the drug company Pfizer was first launching the erectile dysfunction drug Viagra, it simultaneously helped launch a patient support group called Impotence Anonymous with a donation of A$200,000.[20] Pfizer also funded a giant advertising campaign in Australian newspapers featuring full-page advertisements of unhappy-looking couples—yet the drug company name appeared nowhere on the ad. Instead there were the names of other groups, including Impotence Anonymous. When the media tried to interview Pfizer about the advertisements, the staff declined interviews, referring journalists instead to the new chief of Impotence Australia, who claimed his tiny group was independent from Pfizer but admitted that he 'could understand that people may have a feeling that this is a front for Pfizer'.

Sadly, we need to be highly sceptical of statements and materials coming from patient support groups or medical foundations that rely on corporate sponsorship, and we need to ask tough questions about who those sponsors are and what influence they wield. Next time a patient advocate makes an enthusiastic comment about a new drug in a television news report, ask yourself: 'Who else is profiting here?' You could even ask the advocate, if you can find them: 'Does this patient group accept sponsorship from drug companies?' And bear in mind that sponsorship is not just about hard cash—the influence of drug giants comes in many forms. Sometimes a patient group's website is set up or maintained with drug company support. Often the advisory committee for a medical foundation includes doctors with close financial ties to the drug companies. Sometimes health consumer groups' annual dinners are sponsored by drug companies, and sometimes the media activities of medical foundations are handled by the same public relations companies that work closely with the drug companies.

Clearly many of the people connected with patient groups are hard-working and dedicated, determined to get more attention for their particular disease, and committed to fighting for safer and more effective and affordable treatments. Some groups take a big proportion of their support from drug companies, others take just a little, and some take nothing. Groups like Health Action International, based in the Netherlands, are an example of a consumer advocacy group that takes no drug company sponsorship and spends a good deal of time explaining why other groups should also reduce their reliance on such money. Whether or not groups should accept funding is a complex and controversial question and one that is receiving more and more attention around the world. For the moment, though, it will pay to ask: 'Does this patient group or medical foundation accept sponsorship from drug companies?'

EXAMPLE 3
Private for-profit medical corporations

One day, during the northern autumn of 2002 in a small Californian town not far from San Francisco, a large team of FBI officers raided a regional hospital. They seized documents from offices relating to the work of two leading heart surgeons who'd performed thousands of procedures on patients. The FBI was acting on allegations that the surgeons had been performing

Be wary of unnecessary care

unnecessary heart operations in order to maximise their profits. As it turned out, the hospital was part of a giant national chain—Tenet Healthcare—which was one of the biggest private hospital chains in the world.[21]

One of the whistleblowers alleging unnecessary care was a priest who had seen one of the surgeons some time before. The surgeon had recommended urgent heart surgery but, because the priest had pressing business in another town, he had not been able to undergo the operation straightaway. The priest's suspicions started to be raised when he was told by other heart specialists that he did not in fact need the recommended surgery at all. After unsuccessfully complaining to the management at the hospital, the priest decided to inform the authorities.

By the following year, while the FBI investigations continued, more than eighty patients had filed a lawsuit alleging that they had undergone unnecessary heart procedures, including tests and operations, at the Californian hospital. The allegations suggested that some of the people who had undergone procedures had no heart problems at all, that heart operations were being driven by the push for higher profits, and that in a small number of cases patients had even died as a result.

Four years later, the case was finally settled, with the company having to pay out an extraordinary US$500 million.

By then almost 800 patients were involved, one of the biggest-ever cases of unnecessary surgery. In a separate settlement, the same company had to pay almost a billion dollars for overcharging Medicare, one of the publicly funded insurance systems in the United States. In regard to the Medicare case, the company did not admit wrongdoing, instead referring to billing errors. More broadly, the company says there have been changes to management and the corporate culture since the heart surgery scandal occurred.[22]

While this case is an extreme example, it is not uncommon that private for-profit health care corporations are caught out rorting the system. In 2000, hospital giant Columbia/HCA paid out US$745 million for overbilling, and in 2001, a joint venture owned by a Japanese and an American drug company had to pay out almost US$900 million for giving kickbacks to doctors for prescribing expensive drugs.[23]

In Australia, where the publicly funded Medicare system has remained strong, the same level of scandal and corruption has not yet emerged, but with a growing private for-profit health sector, wariness is required. For many years Australian health authorities have been fighting to rein in entrepreneurial doctors who see too many patients and conduct too many procedures. However, proving that a patient has undergone unnecessary care can be very difficult, and health authorities have only had very limited success.

The big change in Australia in recent years has been the emergence of giant private for-profit companies, which have bought up local GP clinics across the country—and in some cases testing laboratories and other health services as well.

The fundamental problem with these 'vertically integrated' companies is that there is a strong incentive for doctors to refer their patients within the same company, thereby generating more profits for the company owners. Health authorities have been concerned about the practice but, with Australian governments at both state and federal levels supporting the move towards more privatisation, there has been limited investigation into what this means for patients. One thing you can do is ask questions like: 'Does a company own this medical centre?' and 'Does the company that owns this centre also own the pathology or radiology centres to which you are referring me?'

Conclusion
Who else is profiting here?

For better or worse, the profit motive is widespread within the health and medical industry. Whether you are seeing surgeons or naturopaths, physiotherapists or psychiatrists, in private practice the more often these practitioners see you, and the more things they do to you, the more money they tend to make. These days, to make matters worse, more and more health professionals are working inside large private companies, which regard you and your health problems primarily as a chance to maximise their profits—their duties to shareholders dictate this. And as we have seen, on top of all that, the influence of large profit-driven drug and device manufacturers on doctors and patient groups is widespread. In many cases your health *will* profit from what your doctor or herbalist recommends, creating a win-win all round. But too often you will be prescribed a test or treatment that will profit someone else a lot more than you.

More questions about who else is profiting

Who else is profiting here?
- What are your links with drug companies (or device companies, or complementary medicine companies)?
- Do you disclose all your financial interactions with companies including drug companies?
- Have you considered disentangling yourself from your financial conflicts of interest?
- Does this patient group or medical foundation accept sponsorship from drug companies?
- Does a company own this medical centre?
- Does the company that owns this centre also own the pathology or radiology centres to which you are referring me?
- Who has funded this study?
- Are there any studies or research not funded by drug companies or other for-profits?

Ten

What can I do to help myself?

It can be a mistake to hand over total responsibility for your health care to doctors or any other health professionals. It may lead you to having treatments you don't want or to missing out on treatments you might have wanted to try. It is important to take an active role yourself, wherever possible. Communicating with health professionals is a two-way process, and you need to do your bit by making sure you describe your symptoms, concerns and expectations as clearly as possible. It is up to you to ask questions about your care, and to encourage your health professional to talk to you in language that you understand. It is especially important to take an active role if you have ongoing health problems requiring long-term management, such as diabetes or arthritis. People with chronic conditions like these fare better if they are well informed and doing all they can to control the problem themselves. As well, you can reduce the risk of many common health problems and diseases by being physically active, eating better and probably also eating less. Many people could also benefit from drinking less alcohol. These measures can also help if you already have health problems. Taking some responsibility for your own health can make a real difference.

The pain and swelling in his right hand was excruciating. It was interfering not just with his work but also his ability to do everyday tasks, whether unlocking the front door or opening a bottle of juice. But Jerome Groopman didn't rush into having an operation when it was suggested by a surgeon. That's because Dr Groopman knows only too well of the need for caution when treatments are being recommended. Not only is he a highly respected doctor himself, but he is also an expert on the types of mistakes that doctors can make.

Dr Groopman eventually saw six hand surgeons and was given four different opinions about what was wrong and what should be done about it. He questioned each surgeon closely. If he didn't understand what he was being told, he kept asking questions until he did.

Dr Groopman's quest for the best treatment for his aching hand is described in his book, *How Doctors Think*, which includes many examples of patients being given the wrong diagnosis or treatment.[1] One of the book's main messages is the importance of asking questions and making sure that you understand what you are being told. Not everyone is in Dr Groopman's privileged position, able to afford six different specialists. Nor do we all have the medical knowledge to grill surgeons in great detail. But there's no doubt that most of us could do far more when it comes to asking questions of our doctors.

Many people want more information

Communication is a two-way process, after all. Studies have shown that many people are unhappy with their doctors' communication skills and wish to be given more information. For example, doctors often don't ask their patients if they have any questions.[2] But these sorts of findings are not only a reflection upon doctors. They also suggest that patients could do more to ensure that doctors clearly understand their problems, what information they want and other expectations that they may have of their consultation or treatment.

Many patients are reluctant to ask questions. This is understandable—it can sometimes be very confronting and difficult to ask questions of doctors, especially if they do not take steps to encourage it, or are in a rush or do not seem approachable. It can be particularly daunting if you are unwell and feeling vulnerable or overwhelmed by being in an alien environment like a hospital. As well, some patients do not see it as their role to ask questions—they expect the doctor to fix their problems. But it can be a mistake to sit back and hand over control for your health care.

The first example in this chapter gives plenty of practical tips on how to become more involved in decisions about your health care, as well as some ideas about how to ask the sort of questions that may make a difference to your well-being. These techniques are particularly important for people with long-term health problems, such as diabetes. In countries right around the world, health professionals are recognising the importance of helping patients to play a more active role in managing such conditions. The

Take the initiative

buzzword used to describe this approach is 'self-management'. If you have a chronic health problem, the second example demonstrates why it's so important you find out about this approach. It could add years to your life, as well as life to your years.

Many of the factors that influence our health are outside the control of any one person. As an individual, it can seem that there's not much you can do about the threats posed by bird flu or global warming, for example. But for many common health problems, there is plenty that you can do, both to reduce your risk of getting them in the first place or, if you already are affected, to stop your condition getting worse. Many of us could do much more to ensure that we and our families follow healthy lifestyles.

In the third example you will see that there are many reasons why you can't leave it up to doctors or other health professionals to suggest you make these sorts of changes. You may need to take the initiative, raising such issues yourself. If you ask 'What changes could I make to my lifestyle to help my health?', you might be surprised by just how much you can do.

EXAMPLE 1

Take responsibility for your health

You can't afford not to take responsibility for your health

The phrase 'follow doctor's orders' says so much. It is a reminder that not so long ago, most people expected their doctors to tell them what to do if they were sick. But it's a phrase that is increasingly seen as old-fashioned and unhelpful. And even in the old days, when doctors tended to be more authoritarian, patients often didn't follow their orders or take their medicines as directed.

In general, people are much more likely to do something if they've been involved in the decision about what should be done, and the same is true when people are seeking health care. You are much more likely to get effective care—to take your medications properly, for example—if you are involved in making decisions about it. There is also some evidence to suggest that patients who ask questions end up doing better after treatment.[3] According to the Australian National Health and Medical Research Council, patients who are given a basic information sheet before surgery are less likely to have complications afterwards, more likely to get home quickly, and have less need for pain relief.[4] Patients are also more likely to be satisfied with their care if they have been involved in making decisions about it.

In medical schools around the world, the doctors of tomorrow are being taught about the importance of involving patients in a partnership when making decisions about their care. As mentioned above, this is partly because it is more likely to lead to better results. But it's also about acknowledging that patients have rights. It is their right to have a say in what is going to happen to them and their bodies. But, as that old saying goes, with rights come responsibilities. You also have to be prepared to do your bit. This means making sure that you communicate clearly about your situation, your concerns, and what you want out of the consultation—whether you are seeing a doctor, naturopath or physiotherapist.

You can't expect health professionals to be mind-readers. You can help them by being very clear yourself, whether you are describing your medical history, your symptoms, or how your problem is affecting you. For example, it is very common for people to tell doctors they are feeling tired, so it can often be difficult for doctors to distinguish between the tiredness which is often just part of life and the type of tiredness which might suggest an underlying health problem. Instead of just saying you feel tired, for example, think about how to explain this in a more meaningful way. Before you get to the doctor's surgery, ask yourself questions like these: 'When did I start feeling this tired?' and 'How is it affecting my life?' Are you having to take time off work, for example? Are there any other things going on in your life that might explain it? Is there some disruption in the household, for example? Has it become more noticeable since you started taking any medications? Or you might consider keeping a diary to monitor your symptoms and how they change over time.

Remember that no one knows your body like you do. You know what feels normal for you and what does not. You know how much you drink, what you eat, and how often you exercise. You also know what's important to you—what risks you might be prepared to tolerate during treatment and which ones are unacceptable. You have to help your doctor understand what is going on for you and what is important to you. Doctors are like anyone else—they can leap to assumptions about you and your health problem on the basis of how you look or behave, and sometimes these assumptions may be quite incorrect. You have to help them to become well informed about you. If you have any particular cultural or spiritual beliefs which may be relevant, you need to make sure that the doctor understands these.

One area where this is particularly important is your family's medical history. The types of health problems that your parents and siblings have experienced, and possibly even your grandparents, can have an important bearing on your own likelihood of developing other problems. Providing your doctor with an accurate record of the family's medical history will help them do their job better.

Another critical area is around medication use. It's vital that every health professional you are seeing knows exactly what medicines you are taking, and in what doses. Don't make the common mistake of not including complementary products: it is just as important that you mention these. It can help to write down all the medicines you are taking, even vitamins or other such supplements. Similarly, it's important your doctor has a good understanding of your own medical history. You can't assume that they know everything they need to know from your medical records, which may be incomplete, especially if you have moved around and seen a lot of different doctors over the years.

Dr Jerome Groopman also advises that patients question their doctors about what possibilities they are considering when working out your diagnosis. He says this encourages doctors to think beyond the most obvious or likely ones. Another way to focus doctors' attention is by asking yourself what body parts are near where your pain or symptoms are occurring. 'What we say to a physician and how we say it sculpts his [or her] thinking. That includes not only our answers but our questions,' says Dr Groopman.[5]

He also suggests asking very detailed questions about any treatment being recommended. We've explained in previous chapters why this is so important: you can't assume that the potential benefits of any treatment will outweigh the harms. He says if a surgeon mentions a possible complication, you should ask how often it happens. If a surgeon talks about pain or discomfort from an operation, ask exactly what this is like and how it might affect you, including your ability to care for yourself or do your usual work after the operation.

Dr Groopman's own story also illustrates the importance of asking exactly what to expect from any procedure or treatment. When he finally settled on having hand surgery, he expected to regain 100 per cent use of his hand—to be back to normal, in other words. He was disappointed that, after surgery, his hand was only about 80 per cent of its old self. It was only after the operation, when talking to other surgeons, that he realised this was actually a good outcome and probably the best that could have been expected. Which just goes to show that it's easy even for an expert like Dr Groopman to neglect asking an important question.

Of course, it's easy to forget to ask some questions, so it can help to jot these down before your consultation or as they come to mind. You may also consider keeping a diary to record your symptoms and progress, and to monitor how they change over time. It can also be useful to write down the important points made in a consultation, or ask if you can tape it, or bring a friend or family member to jog your memory. Ask for written information that you can take away to consider when there is more time. This is especially important when bad news is involved. It's very difficult to take in information when you are shocked or upset, and peoples' memories of what they've been told under these circumstances are often mistaken.

Good communication is not just asking more questions. It's also about understanding the answers that you get. You are entitled to be given information in a way that you understand, so if what you are being told isn't clear, it's up to you to let the doctor know. If English is not your first language, ask for an interpreter to help you during the consultation.

There are many ways of conveying medical information, and doctors often overestimate peoples' skills in understanding numbers and concepts such as percentages or probability. Telling someone they have a 10 per cent chance of suffering a side effect from a treatment is the same as saying that one in ten people will suffer a side effect from treatment. Similarly, if you are told that a treatment has a 30 per cent chance of success, this also means that the treatment does not work 70 per cent of the time. Many people will respond differently to the same likelihood of something occurring, depending upon how it is put to them. And different people are helped by different techniques for conveying such information: some find it easier to grasp percentages; others prefer to have the information presented in a pie chart or graph. You can ask for information to be presented in a way that makes sense to you.

Wherever possible, it's advisable to try to get a handle on the probability of something occurring. General terms—such as a side effect being uncommon—can be very misleading. Studies have shown that when doctors say something is rare, what they mean by this is often completely different to what patients understand 'rare' to be. You need to make sure you and your doctor are speaking the same language.

Doctors, for all their years of study, are like anyone else: they're a varied bunch. Some will be comfortable with you asking questions and will actively encourage this. Some will not. Some may make you feel quite awkward about it. Wherever possible, it's worth trying to find a doctor who you feel comfortable with and who allows you to ask the questions on your mind. Experts in medical communication have suggested that doctors should:

- have the ability to communicate complex information using non-technical language
- tailor the amount and pace of information to your needs

- be prepared to draw diagrams to help you understand the issues
- create an environment in which you feel comfortable asking questions
- give you time to take in the information
- encourage your involvement in decision making.[6]

They also suggest that, at the end of consultations, doctors give a quick summary of what's happened, to help make sure you understand what's been said. But this is also useful advice for patients. At the end of any consultation, try summing up what's happened and what you expect to happen next. That gives an opportunity for any misunderstandings to be corrected, and for you to identify any areas where more information is needed. You might also want to ask: 'Have I explained my symptoms, concerns and expectations clearly?' and 'Is there anything about my medical history or my family's medical history that you need to know?'

EXAMPLE 2
Managing chronic conditions

Health services around the world are going through a major readjustment. In the past, they were largely designed to cope with acute problems, such as a serious injury or illness requiring immediate treatment.

But the world has changed. People are living longer, and are often living for many years with chronic health problems associated with growing older, such as arthritis. The success of some medical treatments—such as keeping people with heart disease alive longer—means that many are now surviving illnesses that once might have killed them. In addition, our modern lifestyles, which make it too easy for people to be physically inactive, are contributing to a rise in long-term problems, such as diabetes.

Become involved in your care

When people have a broken arm, it is treated and fixed, but many people with chronic conditions will never be cured. They have to learn to live with their condition and to manage it as best they can, hopefully preventing it from getting any worse. But many health services and professionals are stuck in the past, still focused on treating acute problems and struggling to provide appropriate long-term support for people with chronic conditions.

Dr Christine Connors is a GP and public health physician who heads the Preventable Chronic Disease Strategy of Australia's Northern Territory government. She has been at the forefront of efforts to reorient the health system towards looking after people with long-term problems and says the changes can be difficult and confronting for both patients and health professionals. 'It's a whole new way of thinking about how you work,' she explains. 'This is not the stuff that we're taught at medical school and unfortunately it's still not the stuff that we're taught at medical schools. We mostly think and practise within an acute paradigm, in which a person asks for our help when they're sick and they mostly have a single cause of their illness.

'We're the experts and say, "This is your problem, I'll fix you." The patients can be passive. We fix them and they go on their way.' By contrast, Dr Connors says, effective chronic care requires a team of health professionals and patients working together over the long term. 'We can't cure them, and that sets up a huge amount of frustration for health staff as well as our patients,' she says. 'We try to tell them what to do, which is what we're used to doing for an acute illness, and it doesn't work.'[7] What patients with chronic problems need from health professionals is support to enable them to take control of their problem. They not only need to own the problem but also the solution. Involving people in making decisions about their care is even more important when they require ongoing care, perhaps over many years.

Self-management programs are designed to do exactly that. If you have a chronic condition like diabetes or heart disease, it is worth finding out more about these programs. Usually in the form of short courses, which can be run face-to-face or over the Internet, typically they teach you: about your condition, how to manage symptoms such as pain and fatigue, how to problem-solve, the benefits of physical activity, how to navigate the health system and to communicate effectively with health professionals, to be aware of your own behaviour and its impact on your condition, and how to manage any related emotional or psychological issues. Such courses have been shown to help improve some patients' well-being and control of their symptoms and, in some cases, to prevent their condition getting worse.

But you can't necessarily rely on your doctor or health service to put you in touch with a self-management course. Studies in Australia and overseas have shown that many doctors and other health professionals are reluctant to refer people to them.[8] Doctors may not know about them, or may be sceptical about their impact, or may resist new ways of doing things or losing 'control' of their patients. Whatever the reason, don't wait to be told about self-management courses. Ask.

The courses may not suit everyone—they take some effort and commitment. But people who've done them often say things like, 'Before the course, my heart problems had control of my life, and now I have control of my heart problems.' Researchers at the Stanford Patient Education Research Center in the United States have been at the forefront of developing self-management courses, and you can find many other courses by searching on the web (you may like to start your search at: <patienteducation.stanford. edu/programs>). If you are dealing with a long-term health issue, you might consider asking your doctor: 'Are there any self-management programs for my problem?' and 'Are there any changes I could make to my lifestyle that might help?'

EXAMPLE 3
Protecting your health

When researchers objectively study what people eat (and other aspects of their lifestyle), and compare their findings with how people *say* they eat (and so on), they find a few surprises. It turns out that most people think they eat better than they really do.[9] We also eat more than we think, and

Make lifestyle changes

tend to think we get more exercise than we really do. And many of us also don't realise that we're drinking more alcohol than is good for us.

In other words, most people could benefit their health by making even relatively minor changes to their daily lives—for example, by eating an extra few serves of vegetables, or by walking to the shops instead of driving, or by having a glass of water with dinner instead of soft drink or a few beers. At some level, many of us already know this. We just need someone to prompt us to make changes.

Doctors are ideally placed to give this prompt. Studies show that doctors have quite a lot of influence over patients. If a doctor suggests we stop smoking or try to stop drinking so much, it often leads to people making changes in their lives. One of the authors of this book gave up smoking cigarettes for good after a doctor simply wrote 'stop smoking' on a little scrap of paper in the surgery. The trouble is that many doctors do not raise these issues.

They can feel awkward about raising issues that seem very personal and they may not know how to do it. They may have problems themselves—like drinking too much—and this can make them less likely to recognise such problems in others. Or they may not want to offend or upset patients. They may have a full waiting room and feel they don't have the time to spend talking to you about how to make changes to your lifestyle. As well, the health system traditionally has not rewarded doctors for encouraging patients to make changes. A surgeon gets paid far more for performing surgery to treat obesity or heart disease than a GP gets paid for taking the time to sit down and talk with patients about how to reduce their risk of developing these problems in the first place.

Don't wait for your doctor to ask about your lifestyle. Bring up the issue yourself. If your doctor can't help, other health professionals might be able to. Psychologists, naturopaths, dietitians, nurses—many different professionals have skills and expertise in helping people to change their behaviour.

While making changes to your lifestyle can help reduce your risk of developing many diseases and health problems, it's also important to ask about what lifestyle changes might help if you already have an illness. If you've had surgery for heart disease, for example, it's vital that you make physical activity part of your daily routine. It can help your recovery and reduce your risk of further heart problems. Eating well and being physically active can also help you cope better with demanding treatments, such as those for cancer.

Of course, all this is often easier said than done. Many of us are stuck in bad habits and unhealthy routines. It can be difficult to make long-lasting change, especially when the modern environment is often so conducive to unhealthy lifestyles. Long working hours, our reliance on cars and computers, the ready availability and widespread promotion of alcohol and fattening foods, time pressures—all of these factors can contribute to people eating too much and moving too little.

It can help to think about these things as an environmental health issue. This focus can take away the blame and guilt, which can be so counterproductive for anyone trying to make lifestyle changes. It also helps you develop long-lasting solutions, rather than quick fixes such as diets, which rarely work long term and may even make the problem worse. So instead of saying 'I must drink less' or 'I must eat less', work out ways of changing your environment to help you do this. It might mean stocking your kitchen cupboards with mineral water rather than alcohol. It might mean buying fruit, rather than sweet, fatty snacks, for those times you crave a nibble. It might mean leaving your walking shoes by the front door, to prompt you to have that morning walk.

When seeing a health professional, you may want to ask: 'Do you have any suggestions for how I could improve my diet? and 'Do you have any ideas about how I could become more physically active?' Many people might also benefit from asking: 'Do you think I drink too much alcohol?'

Conclusion
What can I do to help myself?

Many of us have become too reliant on the health and medical industry. Rather than asking what we can do to help ourselves, we turn to doctors seeking a quick fix. It's often easier to ask for a prescription than to ask what we can do to help ourselves.

And yet, taking more responsibility for your own health is likely to bring many benefits. It may lead to real improvements in your well-being as well as saving you from unnecessary and possibly even harmful tests and treatments. As well, there is much evidence that when people feel some sense of control over their lives, this is good for their health. Taking some responsibility for your health could have many positive spin-offs.

It's not easy. It requires us to make changes to how we behave when consulting with doctors or other health professionals. We have to learn to communicate more effectively, and be very clear about what we want or expect from our care. It also requires many of us to make changes to the way we live. It's far better to prevent health problems occurring in the first place than to end up needing tests and treatments that bring their own risks. If you are already unwell or have a health problem, making changes to your lifestyle can often do as much good as taking medicine or having other treatments.

Remember, your health is too important to leave it in someone else's hands.

More questions about what you can do

What can I do to help myself?

- Have I explained my symptoms, concerns and expectations clearly?
- Is there anything about my medical history or my family's medical history that you need to know?
- Have you got a note of all the medicines and complementary health products I am taking?
- Can you explain more precisely what you mean by the probability of side effects?
- Can you explain this in a diagram?
- Can I have an interpreter?
- Can I bring a friend or family member to the consultation?
- Are there any self-management programs for my problem?
- Are there any changes I could make to my lifestyle that might help?
- Are there any lifestyle changes that I could make instead of taking medicine or having surgery?
- Do you have any suggestions for how I could improve my diet?
- Do you have any ideas about how I could become more physically active?
- Do you think I drink too much alcohol?

Conclusion

Developing a healthy scepticism

When you are sick or out of sorts, it is easy to feel vulnerable. You want to be able to trust the person to whom you turn for help, whether they are a nurse, a neurosurgeon or a naturopath. One of the problems with asking lots of questions of your carer is that it is easy to give the impression of not fully trusting them.

We all need to move beyond this mindset, however, whether we are doctors or patients. Asking questions needs to be seen as an essential and valid part of seeking health care. As you have read in this book, there are so many reasons why we all need to be much more proactive in doing this. To put it bluntly, if you don't, your health and well-being may suffer. It is important that you not only ask questions of those charged with providing your health care but also of yourself. You may benefit from examining some of your own belief systems and habits, or from questioning your own role in protecting that precious resource known as your health.

Difficult though it can be to question your doctor, in some ways that is the easy part. Getting answers and working out what to do with that information can be much more challenging. Often, the more we learn about a disease or a treatment, the more uncertain things become. It is rarely the case that there are clear, simple answers to all of our questions. Frequently there is a great deal of doubt about the best way to treat an illness, or even whether to treat it at all, what side effects might arise, how likely they are and how serious they might be. Often there is a range of options, with different potential risks or benefits, and we can face tough decisions about what to do.

As the examples in this book have shown, patients and health professionals often have to make decisions in the absence of good evidence. Often there is a lack of reliable information about the merits of various tests and treatments because the relevant, high quality research has not been done. One way patients can contribute to the development of more reliable information is to participate in clinical trials. Not all these trials are worthwhile: sometimes studies are conducted to help companies market their products, rather than to answer important questions about the merits of tests and treatments. However, if you can be sure the research is being done by independent researchers and for the right reasons, you may wish to be involved. Your participation may help lead to improvements in the care you and others receive.

While we have focused in this book on what sorts of questions to ask, and spent a little time listing a few reliable websites for those readers wanting to do more research, we have not devoted much time to examining how to use the information you get and how to make those tough decisions that follow. Obviously, when there are big decisions to be made, we would urge you to try to talk to your doctors and other carers, your family and friends as much as you can about the pros and cons. If the current trends towards patient empowerment continue, it will not be long before there are paid professionals who will specialise in being able to help you make the best decisions for your situation. Already some health systems offer services where you can call a nurse or other professional and get some timely advice. Sometimes our doctors already fulfil that role, but they do not always have the ability or time to sit with us and help navigate through the sea of evidence and options to find the best route.

As you will have no doubt gathered, many of the examples in this book show the health and medical industry in a negative light. It should be clear, though, that alongside all those negatives, there are many, many positive examples of treatments that save lives or restore quality of life. The aim of this book is not to frighten people away from care they need. Our goal is to encourage people to be healthy sceptics, so we can all avoid useless, unnecessary and dangerous tests and treatments. As we stated in the introduction, we want to share the scepticism we've gained as journalists through our years of listening to doctors and other health professionals, and through reading literally thousands of academic papers documenting the downsides of modern medicine.

Ironically, there is not yet overwhelming evidence to support our claim that asking questions and becoming more informed can improve your health.[1] We suspect, however, that as more researchers study this field, the more likely it is that this will be shown to be so. Rather than damaging trust between patient and doctor, we believe that a more questioning approach can enrich that relationship, leading to better outcomes for everyone. A dose of healthy scepticism may, as they say, be just what the doctor ordered.

Recommended reading

Websites

Bandolier (United Kingdom)
www.jr2.ox.ac.uk/bandolier
Oxford scientists provide regular updates on the latest evidence about health and medical treatments.

BMJ Best Treatments (United Kingdom)
besttreatments.bmj.com/btuk/home.jsp
This site from the British Medical Journal Publishing Group aims to help patients and doctors work together by providing both with the best research evidence about treatments.

Cochrane Database of Systematic Reviews
www.cochrane.org/reviews
The Cochrane Collaboration, an international group working to improve the evidence base of health care, provides this electronic library of its summaries of the evidence for various tests and treatments. Australians have free access through the National Institute of Clinical Studies: www.nhmrc.gov.au/nics/asp/index.asp?

DIPEx (United Kingdom)

www.dipex.org

The Database of Individual Patient Experiences website has a wide variety of peoples' personal experiences of health and illness. You can watch, listen to or read their interviews, and find reliable information on treatment choices and where to get support. This not-for-profit organisation is funded by the UK Department of Health and other British health groups.

DISCERN (United Kingdom)

www.discern.org.uk

University of Oxford researchers have developed this website to help the general public and health professionals better assess the quality of health advice and information.

Health News Review (United States)

www.healthnewsreview.org

The Foundation for Informed Medical Decision Making in the United States provides analyses of the quality of media coverage of treatments, tests and procedures.

Hitting the Headlines (United Kingdom)

www.library.nhs.uk

English researchers provide a rapid analysis of the evidence behind media stories of new tests, treatments and procedures. Many of these stories also appear in Australian outlets.

James Lind Library

www.jameslindlibrary.org

The James Lind Library provides a weath of useful resources about the evidence basis of health care.

Media Doctor Australia

www.mediadoctor.org.au

A group from Newcastle analyse the quality of media stories about medical tests and treatments.

Media Doctor Canada
www.mediadoctor.ca
A sister site to the Australian group, providing similar analysis of media stories.

Patient Decision Aids (Canada)
www.decisionaid.ohri.ca
A quality-controlled list of many decision aids from around the world, produced by the Ottawa Health Research Institute.

Sydney Health Decision Group (Australia)
www.health.usyd.edu.au/shdg/
Academics at the University of Sydney are developing decision aids and other tools to help patients and health professionals incorporate evidence into their decision making.

Books

Marcia Angell, *The Truth About the Drug Companies*, Scribe, Melbourne, 2005.

Imogen Evans, Hazel Thorton and Iain Chalmers, *Testing Treatments: better research for better healthcare*, The British Library, London, 2006. (This book is freely available in electronic format from the James Lind Library at http://www.jameslindlibrary.org)

Atul Gawande, *Complications: A surgeon's notes on an imperfect science*, Profile Books, London, 2002.

Jerome Groopman, *How Doctors Think*, Scribe, Melbourne, 2007.

Les Irwig, Judy Irwig, Lyndal Trevena and Melissa Sweet, *Smart Health Choices: Making sense of health advice*, Hammersmith Press, London, 2008.

Ray Moynihan and Alan Cassels, *Selling Sickness: How drug companies are turning us all into patients*, Allen & Unwin, Sydney, 2005.

Bill Runciman, Alan Merry and Merrilyn Walton, *Safety and Ethics in Health Care: A guide to getting it right*, Ashgate, Hampshire, 2007.

Merrilyn Walton, *Well Being: How to get the best treatment from your doctor*, Pluto Press, Sydney, 2002.

Notes

Introduction

1   J. Irwig, L. Irwig, and M. Sweet, *Smart Health Choices*, Allen & Unwin, Sydney, 1999; R. Moynihan and A. Cassels, *Selling Sickness: How the drug companies are turning us all into patients*, Allen & Unwin, Sydney, 2005; R. Moynihan, *Too Much Medicine?*, ABC Books, Sydney, 1998.

Chapter 1

1   This story is based on the article by S. Birnbaum, 'CT scanning: Too much of a good thing', *BMJ*, vol. 334, May 2007, p. 1006.
2   S. Amis et al., 'American College of Radiology White Paper on radiation dose in medicine', *Journal of the American College of Radiology*, vol. 4, no. 5, May 2007, pp. 272–84.
3   J. Iglehart, 'The new era of medical imaging: Progress and pitfalls', *New England Journal of Medicine*, vol. 354, no. 26, Jun. 2006, pp. 2822–8.
4   S. Amis et al., 'American College of Radiology White Paper', pp. 272–84.

5   L. Berlin, 'Communicating radiology results', *The Lancet*, vol. 367, Feb. 2006, pp. 373–5.

6   K. Petrie et al., 'Effect of providing information about normal test results on patients' reassurance: Randomised controlled trial', *BMJ*, vol. 334, no. 7589, Feb. 2007, p. 352.

7   S. Amis et al., 'American College of Radiology White Paper', pp. 272–84.

8   The American College of Radiology has a site explaining exposure at <www.radiologyinfo.org/en/safety [29 May 2007].

9   S. Amis et al., 'American College of Radiology White Paper', pp. 272–84.

10   Commonwealth Scientific and Industrial Research Organisation, 'Safer CT scans for children', press release, <www.csiro.au/news/psw0.html> [8 November 2007]

11   P. Hall, 'Effect of low doses of ionizing radiation in infancy on cognitive function in adulthood: Swedish population based cohort study', *BMJ*, vol. 328, no. 7430, Jan. 2004, p. 19.

12   Office of the Auditor-General of Ontario, 'Hospitals: Management and use of diagnostic imaging equipment', 2006 <www.auditor.on.ca/en/reports_en/en06/306en06.pdf> [7 November 2007].

13   J. Iglehart, 'The new era of medical imaging', pp. 2822–8.

14   J. Iglehart, 'The new era of medical imaging—progress and pitfalls', pp. 2822–8.

15   'Risk: Think twice on CT scans', *Australian Doctor*, 27 Jul. 2007, p. 1.

16   T. Wilt and I. Thompson, 'Clinically localised prostate cancer', *BMJ*, vol. 333, Nov. 2006, pp. 1102–6.

17   This comes from an online decision aid produced by the organisation Preferred Care, 'Should I have a prostate-specific antigen (PSA) test to screen for prostate cancer?', <www.healthwise.net/preferredcare/Content/StdDocument.aspx?DOCHWID=aa38144&SECHWID=aa38144-Intro> [7 Nov 2007]

18   'False positive PSA is associated with increased worry', *BMJ*, vol. 330, Mar. 2005. Note: Some of the false positive men also ultimately feel like they 'dodged a bullet', according to this paper.

19   Wilt and Thompson, 'Clinically localised prostate cancer', pp. 1102–6.

20   H.G. Welch, L.M. Schwartz and S. Woloshin, 'Prostate specific antigen levels in the United States: Implications of various definitions for abnormal', *Journal of the National Cancer Institute*, vol. 97, no. 15, Aug. 2005, pp. 1132–7.

21   This evidence will be cited in chapter 3.

22   The International Network of Cholesterol Skeptics has a home page at <www.thincs.org> [7 November 2007]

23   R. Moynihan and A. Cassels, *Selling Sickness*, Allen & Unwin, Sydney, 2005, chapter 1.

24   Birnbaum, 'CT scanning: Too much of a good thing'.

Chapter 2

1   R. Moynihan, *Too Much Medicine?*, ABC Books, Sydney, 1998.

2   J. Tanne, 'ADHD drugs should carry warning, FDA committee recommends', *BMJ*, vol. 332, Apr. 2006, p. 748.

3   R. Moynihan and A. Cassels, *Selling Sickness*, Allen & Unwin, Sydney, 2005, chapter 4.

4   A. Kazanjian, C. Green and K. Bassett, 'Normal bone mass, aging bodies, marketing of fear: Bone mineral density testing of well women', British Columbia Office of Health Technology Assessment, University of British Colombia, presented at the 93rd annual meeting of the American Sociological Association, held in San Francisco, 21–25 August 1998.

5   Moynihan and Cassels, *Selling Sickness*, chapter 10.

6   This example is based on the references which appear in chapter 4 of Moynihan and Cassels, *Selling Sickness*.

7   This paragraph is informed by S. Okie, 'ADHD in adults', *New England Journal of Medicine*, vol. 345, no. 25, Jun. 2006, pp. 2637–41.

8   S. Nissen, 'ADHD drugs and cardiovascular risk', *New England Journal of Medicine*, vol. 354, no. 14, Apr. 2006, pp. 1445–8.

9   S. Nissen, 'ADHD Drugs and Cardiovascular Risk', pp. 1445–8.

10   <www.fda.gov/ohrms/dockets/ac/06/briefing/2006–4210b_17_01_CV%20labeling%20list.pdf> [8 November 2007].

11   Moynihan and Cassels, *Selling Sickness*, chapter 4.

12   <www.shire.com/shire/financialReports/ar2006/financial.html>
      [8 November 2007].

13   S. Nissen, 'ADHD Drugs and Cardiovascular Risk', pp. 1445–8.

14   <www.australiandoctor.com.au/articles/a7/0c04d7a7.asp>

15   K. Pearce, 'Osteoporosis is a risk factor not a disease', *BMJ*,
      vol. 322, Apr. 2001, p. 862.

16   Moynihan and Cassels, *Selling Sickness*, chapter 8 (much of the
      material on this example is informed by the many references for
      this chapter).

17   G. Sanson, *The Osteoporosis 'Epidemic'*, Penguin, Auckland, 2001.

18   P. Alonso, A. Garcia-Franco, G. Guyatt and R. Moynihan, 'Drugs
      for pre-osteoporosis: prevention or disease-mongery', *BMJ*,
      vol. 336, pp. 126–9.

19   Moynihan and Cassels, *Selling Sickness*, chapter 8.

20   T. Masud and R.M. Francis, 'The increasing use of peripheral
      bone densitometry', *BMJ*, vol. 321, Aug. 2000, pp. 396–8.

21   Pearce, 'Osteoporosis is a risk factor', p. 862.

22   L.D. Gillespie, et al., 'Interventions for preventing falls in the
      elderly', *Cochrane Database of Systematic Reviews*, Issue 4, 1997.

23   Patient information on Fosamax: <www.merck.com/product/usa/
      pi_circulars/f/fosamax/fosamax_onceweekly_ppi.pdf>
      [8 November 2007].

24   This example is based on references in Moynihan and Cassels,
      Selling Sickness, chapter 10.

25   V. Parry, 'The art of branding a condition', *MM&M*, May 2003,
      pp. 43–9.

26   E. Kaschak and L. Tiefer, *A New View of Women's Sexual Problems*,
      The Haworth Press, New York, 2001.

27   Datamonitor, 'Female sexual dysfunction: Prescription drug
      pipeline overview 2007', <www.datamonitor.com/industries/
      research/?pid=DMHC2334> [8 November 2007].

Chapter 3

1   Interview with Simon Chapman, 2007.

2   L. Irwig et al., 'Informed choice for screening: Implications for
     evaluation', *BMJ*, vol. 332, May 2006, pp. 1148–50.

3   Notes on prostate cancer screening will appear in Example 1.

4   Notes on breast cancer screening will appear in Example 2.

5   Notes for this material will appear in Example 3.

6   R. McKenzie et al., 'The news is not all good', *Medical Journal of Australia*, vol. 187, no. 9, Nov. 2007, pp. 507–10.

7   R. McKenzie et al., ' The news is not all good', pp. 507–10.

8   D. Ilic et al., 'Screening for prostate cancer', *Cochrane Collaboration Systematic Review*, art. no.: CD004720 (doi:10.1002/14651858.CD004720.pub2, updated 8 May 2006).

9   McKenzie et al., 'The news is not all good', pp. 507–10.

10   Interview with Simon Chapman, 2007.

11   S. Chapman, 'The hyping of prostate cancer' www.crikey.com.au.

12   S. Chapman, 'The hyping of prostate cancer' www.crikey.com.au.

13   L. Holmberg et al., *New England Journal of Medicine*, vol. 347, Sept. 2002, pp. 781–9.

14   N. Pashayan et al., 'Excess cases of prostate cancer and estimated overdiagnosis associated with PSA testing in East Anglia', *British Journal of Cancer*, vol. 95, Jul. 2006, pp. 401–5.

15   McKenzie et al., ' The news is not all good', pp. 507–10.

16   Interview with Simon Chapman, 2007.

17   P. Gotzsche and M. Nielsen, 'Screening for breast cancer with mammography', *Cochrane Collaboration Systematic Review*, art. no.: CD001877 (doi:10.1002/14651858.CD001877.pub2, updated Jul. 2006).

18   A systematic review is a review of all the best studies, where the results are summarised, giving very strong evidence. Read more about this in chapter 8.

19   H. Moller and E. Davies, 'Commentary: Over-diagnosis in breast cancer screening', *BMJ*, vol. 332, Mar. 2006, pp. 691–2.

20   Gotzsche and Nielsen, 'Screening for breast cancer'.

21   Moller and Davies, 'Commentary: Over-diagnosis', pp. 691–2.

22   J.M. Dixon, *BMJ*, vol. 332, March 2006, pp. 499–500.

23   The University of Sydney, 'Australian screening mammography decision aid trial', <www.mammogram.med.usyd.edu.au> [12 November 2007].

24   Australian screening mammography decision aid trial.

25   Australian screening mammography decision aid trial.

26 PR Web/Newswire press release, 'American Journal of Cardiology to publish SHAPE Task Force Report', 10 Jul. 2006.

27 F. Charatan, 'Cardiologists urge screening of asymptomatic older people', *BMJ*, vol. 333, Jul. 2006, p. 168.

28 <www.shapesociety.org/site/c.iuIRL8MVJxE/b.2804333/k.CE0C/ Partners.htm> [12 November 2007].

29 R. Moynihan and A. Cassels, *Selling Sickness*, Allen & Unwin, Sydney, 2005, chapter 1.

30 United States Preventive Services Task Force, 'Screening for coronary heart disease', Feb. 2004.

31 Coronary calcium scans: Heart scans mired in controversy', <www.mayoclinic.com/print/heart-disease/HB00015/ METHOD=print> [12 November 2007].

32 A. Einstein et al., 'Estimating risk of cancer associated with radiation exposure from 64-slice computed tomography coronary angiography', *Journal of the American Medical Association*, vol. 298, no. 3, Jul. 2007, pp. 317–23.

Chapter 4

1 B.W. Koes, M.W. van Tulder and S. Thomas, 'Clinical review: Diagnosis and treatment of low back pain', *BMJ*, vol. 332, Jun. 2006, pp. 1430–4.

2 B.W. Koes, M.W. van Tulder and S. Thomas, 'Clinical review Diagnosis' pp. 1430–4.

3 W.B. Runciman, M.J. Edmonds and M. Pradhan, 'Setting priorities for patient safety', *Quality and Safety in Health Care*, vol. 11, Jan. 2002, pp. 224–9.

4 P. Little, 'Delayed prescribing: A sensible approach to the management of acute otitis media', *Journal of the American Medical Association*. vol. 296, Sept. 2006, pp. 1290–1.

5 M.M. Rovers et al., 'Antibiotics for acute otitis media: A meta-analysis with individual patient data', *BMJ*, vol. 368, Oct. 2006, pp. 1429–35.

6 R.P. Rietveld, P.J.E. Bindels and G. ter Riet, 'Antibiotics for upper respiratory tract infections and conjunctivitis in primary care', *BMJ*, vol. 333, Aug. 2006, pp. 311–12. H.A. Everitt, P.S. Little and

P.W.F. Smith, 'A randomised controlled trial of management strategies for acute infective conjunctivitis in general practice', *BMJ*, vol. 333, Aug. 2006, p. 321.

7   T.Whelan et al., 'Effect of a decision aid on knowledge and treatment decision making for breast cancer surgery', *Journal of the American Medical Association*, vol. 292, Jul. 2004, pp. 435–41.

8   A. O'Connor, et al., 'Effectiveness of decision aids for people facing health treatment or screening decisions', *Best Evidence Health Care Cochrane Colloquium*, vol. 7, Oct. 1999, Univesità S. Tommaso D'Aquino, p. 79. G. Elwyn et al., 'Developing a quality criteria framework for patient decision aids: Online international Delphi consensus process', *BMJ*, vol. 333, Aug. 2006, p. 417.

Chapter 5

1   A.W. Jørgensen, J. Hilden and P.C. Gøtzsche, 'Research Cochrane reviews compared with industry supported meta-analyses and other meta-analyses of the same drugs: Systematic review', *BMJ*, vol. 333, Oct. 2006, pp. 782–5.

2   G. Bjelakovic et al., 'Review: Mortality in randomized trials of antioxidant supplements for primary and secondary prevention systematic review and meta-analysis', *Journal of the American Medical Association*, vol. 297, Feb. 2007, pp. 842–57.

3   W.C. Willett and M.J. Stampfer, 'Clinical practice: What vitamins should I be taking, doctor?', *New England Journal of Medicine*, vol. 34, Dec. 2001, pp. 1819–24. R.H. Fletcher and K.M. Fairfield, 'Vitamins for chronic disease prevention in adults: Clinical applications', *Journal of the American Medical Association*, vol. 287, Jun. 2002, pp. 3127–9.

4   G. Bjelakovic et al., 'Review: Mortality in randomized trials', pp. 842–57. E.R. Miller III et al., 'Meta-analysis: High-dosage vitamin E supplementation may increase all-cause mortality', *Annals of Internal Medicine*, vol. 142, Jan. 2005, pp. 37–46.

5   M.L. Ancelin et al., 'Non-degenerative mild cognitive impairment in elderly people and use of anticholinergic drugs: Longitudinal cohort study', *BMJ*, vol. 332, Feb. 2006, pp. 455–9.

6   B.A. Briesacher et al., 'The quality of antipsychotic drug prescribing in nursing homes', *Archives of Internal Medicine*, vol. 165, Jun. 2005, pp. 1280–5.

7   A.J. Pelosi, S.V. McNulty and G.A. Jackson, 'Role of cholinesterase inhibitors in dementia care needs rethinking', *BMJ*, vol. 333, Sept. 2006, pp. 491–3.

8   S.M. Jani et al., (for the American College of Cardiology Foundation Guidelines Applied in Practice Steering Committee), 'Sex differences in the application of evidence-based therapies for the treatment of acute myocardial infarction', *Archives of Internal Medicine*, vol. 166, Jun. 2006, pp. 1164–70.

9   S.M. Grundy, 'Should women be offered cholesterol lowering drugs to prevent cardiovascular disease? Yes', *BMJ*, vol. 334, May 2007, p. 982. M. Kendrick, 'Should women be offered cholesterol lowering drugs to prevent cardiovascular disease? No', *BMJ*, vol. 334, May 2007, p. 983.

10 N.P. Stocks, P. Ryan, H. McElroy and J. Allan, 'Statin prescribing in Australia: Socioeconomic and sex differences: A cross-sectional study', *Medical Journal of Australia*, vol. 180, Mar. 2004, pp. 229–31.

Chapter 6

1   B. Runciman, A. Merry and M. Walton, *Safety and Ethics in Health Care: A guide to getting it right*, Ashgate, Aldershot, 2007.

2   E.E. Roughead and J. Lexchin, 'Adverse drug events: Counting is not enough, action is needed', *Medical Journal of Australia*, vol. 184, Apr. 2006, pp. 315–16.

3   S. Motl, E. Timpe and S. Eichner, 'Proposal to improve MedWatch: Decentralized, regional surveillance of adverse drug reactions', *American Journal of Health System Pharmacy*, vol. 61, Sept. 2004, pp. 1840–2.

4   L. Hitchen, 'Adverse drug reactions result in 250 000 UK admissions a year', *BMJ*, vol. 332, May 2006, p. 332.

5   Centers for Disease Control and Prevention, 'Morbidity and mortality weekly report: Infant deaths associated with cough and cold medications—two states, 2005', *Journal of the American Medical Association*, vol. 297, Feb. 2007, pp. 800–1.

6 Institute of Medicine of the National Academies, *The Future of Drug Safety: Promoting and protecting the health of the public*, The National Academies Press, Washington DC, 2006 (available at: <www.nap.edu>).

7 J.R. Stockigt, 'Barriers in the quest for quality drug information: Salutary lessons from TGA-approved sources for thyroid-related medications', *Medical Journal of Australia*, vol. 186, Jan. 2007, pp. 76–9.

8 Australian Government press release, 'Relief for half a million arthritis sufferers: Wooldridge', 1 June 2000 (available at <www. health.gov.au/internet/wcms/publishing.nsf/Content/health-mediarel-yr2000-mw-mw20048.htm>).

9 D.J. Graham, 'COX-2 inhibitors, other NSAIDs, and cardiovascular risk: The seduction of common sense. Editorial', *Journal of the American Medical Association*, vol. 296, Oct. 2006, pp. 1653–6. H.A. Waxman, 'The lessons of Vioxx: Drug safety and sales', *New England Journal of Medicine*, vol. 352, May 2005, pp. 2576–8.

10 J. Avorn, 'Dangerous deception: Hiding the evidence of adverse drug effects', *New England Journal of Medicine*, vol. 355, Nov. 2006, pp. 2169–71. H.A. Waxman, 'The lessons of Vioxx', pp. 2576–8. E.E. Roughead and Lexchin, 'Adverse drug events', pp. 315–16.

11 C. Johnson, 'OxyContin makers admit deception: Addiction danger from painkiller was understated', *Washington Post*, 11 May 2007.

12 J. Feeley and M.F. Cortez, 'US FDA warned Glaxo in 2001 about Avandia marketing', *Bloomberg.com*, 24 May 2007. (available at <www. bloomberg.com/apps/news?pid=newsarchive&sid=awszvyw2rhey>).

13 J. Avorn, 'Dangerous deception', pp. 2169–71.

14 M. Coceani and R. Mariotti, 'Is amiodarone safe in heart failure?', *BMJ*, vol. 332, Feb. 2006, pp. 317–18.

15 T. Gibian, 'Rational drug therapy in the elderly or how not to poison your elderly patients', *Australian Family Physician*, vol. 21, Dec. 1992, pp. 1755–60.

16 M. Chan, F. Nicklason and J.H. Vial, 'Adverse drug events as a cause of hospital admission in the elderly', *Internal Medicine Journal*, vol. 31, May/Jun. 2001, pp. 199–205.

17 E.E. Roughead, B. Anderson and A.L. Gilbert, 'Potentially inappropriate prescribing among Australian veterans and war

widows/widowers', *Internal Medicine Journal,* vol. 37, Jun. 2007, pp. 402–5.

18 C.L. Burgess, C.D.J. Holman and A.G. Satti, 'Adverse drug reactions in older Australians, 1981–2002', *Medical Journal of Australia,* vol. 182, Mar. 2005, pp. 267–70.

19 E.E. Roughead, J.D. Barratt and A.L. Gilbert, 'Medication-related problems commonly occurring in an Australian community setting', *Pharmacoepidemiology and Drug Safety,* vol. 13, Dec. 2003, pp. 83–7.

20 E.E. Roughead, 'Managing adverse drug reactions: Time to get serious', *Medical Journal of Australia,* vol. 182, Mar. 2005, pp. 264–5.

21 R.M. Wilson, W.B. Runciman, R.W. Gibberd et al., 'The quality in Australian health care study', *Medical Journal of Australia,* Nov. 1995, vol. 163, pp. 458–71.

22 B. Runciman, A. Merry and M. Walton, *Safety and Ethics in Health Care: A guide to getting it right,* Ashgate, Aldershot, 2007.

23 B. Runciman et al., *Safety and Ethics in Health Care.*

24 Australian Commission on Safety and Quality in Health Care, '10 tips for safer health care', 2003 <www.health.gov.au/internet/safety/publishing.nsf/Content/10-tips>.

25 A, Tonks, 'Essential oils implicated in prepubertal gynaecomastia', *BMJ,* vol. 334, Feb. 2007, p. 282.

26 S.E. McDowell, J.J. Coleman and R.E. Ferner, 'Systematic review and meta-analysis of ethnic differences in risks of adverse reactions to drugs used in cardiovascular medicine', *BMJ,* vol. 332, May 2006, pp. 1177–81.

Chapter 7

1 Interview with Brian Moynihan (father of co-author Ray Moynihan), 2007.

2 B. Runciman, A. Merry and M. Walton, *Safety and Ethics in Health Care: A guide to getting it right,* Ashgate, Aldershot, 2007.

3 J. Lauer and A. Betran, 'Decision aids for women with a previous caesarean section', *BMJ,* vol. 334, Jun. 2007, pp. 1281–2.

4   S. Green et al., 'Systematic review of randomised controlled trials of interventions for painful shoulder: Selection criteria, outcome assessment, and efficacy', *BMJ*, vol. 316, Jan. 1998, p. 354–60.

5   B. Ejnisman et al., 'Interventions for tears of the rotator cuff in adults', *Cochrane Database of Systematic Reviews*, issue 1, 2004.

6   J.A. Coghlan et al., 'Surgery for rotator cuff disease', *Cochrane Database of Systematic Reviews*, in press.

7   C. Mitchell et al., 'Shoulder pain: Diagnosis and management in primary care,' *BMJ*, vol. 331, Nov. 2005, pp. 1124–8.

8   Despite requests Bill Clark declined to comment.

9   Interview with Rachelle Buchbinder, 2007.

10   T. Diamond et al, 'Clinical Outcomes after acute osteoporotic vertebral fractures: A 2-year non-randomised trial comparing percutaneous vertebroplasty with conservative therapy', *Medical Journal of Australia*, vol. 184, 2006, pp. 113–17.

11   Research for book.

12   R. Buchbinder and R. Osborne, 'Vertebroplasty: A promising but as yet unproven intervention for painful osteoporotic spinal fracures', *Medical Journal of Australia*, vol. 185, 2006, pp. 351–2.

13   Bill Clark is involved in one of the randomised controlled trials.

14   Research for book.

15   A. Shorten et al., 'Making choices for childbirth: Development and testing of a decision-aid for women who have experienced previous caesarean', *Patient Education and Counselling*, vol. 52, 2004, pp. 307–13.

16   A. Montgomery et al., 'Two decision aids for mode of delivery among women with previous caesarean section: Randomised controlled trial', *BMJ*, vol. 334, 23 Jun. 2007, p. 1305.

17   <www.latimes.com/features/health/la-he-induction13aug13, 1,5179922.story?coll=la-headlines-health&ctrack=1&cset=true>.

18   Shorten et al., 'Making choices for childbirth', pp. 307–13.

19   Montgomery et al., 'Two decision aids for mode of delivery', 23 Jun. 2007.

20   Interview with Stephen Leeder, 1997.

Chapter 8

1   P. Perel, I. Roberts, E. Sena, P. Wheble, C. Briscoe, P. Sandercock,
     M. Macleod, L.E. Mignini, J.P. Jayaram and K.S. Khan,
     'Comparison of treatment effects between animal experiments
     and clinical trials: Systematic review', *BMJ*, vol. 334, Jan. 2007,
     p. 197.

2   G. Schwitzer, 'How the media left the evidence out in the cold',
     BMJ, vol. 326, Jun. 2003, pp. 1403–4.

3   J. Hopkins Tanne, 'US television science news is sometimes public
     relations in disguise', *BMJ*, vol. 333, Nov. 2006, p. 1089.

4   G. Schwitzer, 'How the media left the evidence out in the cold'.

5   D. Palmer, 'Regimens for hormone replacement therapy',
     Australian Prescriber, vol. 17, 1994, pp. 130–6.

6   E. Hemminki and K. McPherson, 'Impact of postmenopausal
     hormone therapy on cardiovascular events and cancer: Pooled
     data from clinical trials', *BMJ*, vol. 315, 1997, pp. 149–53.

7   Writing Group for the Women's Health Initiative Investigators,
     'Risks and benefits of estrogen plus progestin in healthy
     postmenopausal women. Principal results from the Women's
     Health Initiative randomized controlled trial', *Journal of the
     American Medical Association*, vol. 288, 2002, pp. 321–33.

8   K. Kerlikowske et al., 'Declines in invasive breast cancer and use
     of postmenopausal hormonal therapy in a screening
     mammography population', *Journal of the National Cancer Institute*,
     2007, vol. 99, pp. 1335–9. The University of Texas MD Anderson
     Cancer Center, media release, 'Decline in breast cancer cases
     likely linked to reduced use of hormone replacement',
     14 Dec. 2006. *Science Daily*, 'Decrease in breast cancer rates likely
     reflect HRT reduction and saturation of mammography', May 5,
     2007, accessed at: <www.sciencedaily.com/releases/2007/05/0705030
     75207.htm>.

9   National Women's Health Network, media release, 'Response to
     the announcement that health risks outweigh benefits for
     combined estrogen plus progestin. Statement of Cynthia Pearson,
     Executive Director, National Women's Health Network', 9 July

2002, Washington DC. For more information about the Network see <www.womenshealthnetwork.org>.

10   S. Bent et al., 'Saw Palmetto for benign prostatic hyperplasia', *New England Journal of Medicine*, vol. 354, Feb. 2006, pp. 557–66.

Chapter 9

1   A. Wazana, 'Physicians and the pharmaceutical industry: Is a gift ever just a gift?' *Journal of the American Medical Association*, vol. 283, Jan. 2000, pp. 373–80. Also see R. Moynihan and A. Cassels, *Selling Sickness*, Allen & Unwin, Sydney, 2005.

2   Theme issue of the *BMJ*, 'Time to untangle doctors from drug companies', vol. 326. 31 May 2003.

3   T. Brennan et al., 'Health industry practices that create conflicts of interest: A policy proposal for academic medical centers', *Journal of the American Medical Association*, vol. 295, Jan. 2006, pp. 429–33.

4   M. Tattersall and I. Kerridge, 'Doctors behaving badly?', *Medical Journal of Australia*, vol. 185, no. 6, Sept. 2006, pp. 299–30.

5   Wazana, 'Physicians and the pharmaceutical industry', pp. 373–80; B. Psaty and D. Rennie, 'Clinical trial investigators and their prescribing patterns: Another dimension to the relationship between physician investigators and the pharmaceutical industry', *Journal of the American Medical Association*, vol. 295, Jun. 2006, pp. 2787–90.

6   M. Day, 'Industry association suspends drug company for entertaining doctors', *BMJ*, vol. 332, Feb. 2006, p. 381.

7   R. Moynihan, 'Roche defends buying lavish meals for doctors at Sydney's restaurants', *BMJ*, vol. 333, Jul. 2006, p. 169.

8   F. Charatan, 'Doctors told to shun rewards from industry as size of payments becomes clear', *BMJ*, vol. 332, Feb. 2006, p. 255.

9   For example, Blackmores was a sponsor of a recent seminar on integrative health care in Byron Bay, Australia, 2007.

10   J. Lexchin et al., 'Pharmaceutical industry sponsorship and research outcome and quality: Systematic review', *BMJ*, vol. 326, May 2003, pp. 1167–70.

11   J. Ross, 'Pharmaceutical company payments to physicians: Early experiences with disclosure laws in Vermont and Minnesota', *Journal of the American Medical Association*, vol. 297, Mar. 2007, pp. 1216–23.

12   Tattersall and Kerridge, 'Doctors behaving badly?', pp. 299–30.

13   <www.healthyskepticism.org>, <www.nofreelunch.org>.

14   Brennan et al., 'Health Industry Practices' pp. 429–33.

15   P. Mansfield, 'Pharma pays the piper: Will Roche call Kidney Health Australia's tune?' <www.crikey.com.au/Politics/20070827-Pharma-pays-the-piper-Will-Roche-call-Kidney-Health-Australias-tune.html> [28 August 2007].

16   'Fundraising and the growth of industry involvement', Health and Social Campaigners News, published by Patient View, Apr. 2004, issue 6.

17   O. Dyer, 'GSK breached marketing code', *BMJ*, vol. 333, Aug. 2006, p. 368.

18   R. Moynihan and A. Cassels, *Selling Sickness*, Allen & Unwin, Sydney, 2005, chapter 4.

19   R. Moynihan, 'Celebrity selling', *BMJ*, vol. 324, June 2002, p. 1342.

20   R. Moynihan, 'Taking the soft option', *Australian Financial Review*, 13 November, 2000, p. 1.

21   Source for this case: F. Charatan, 'FBI investigates cardiac surgeries', *BMJ*, vol. 325, 2002, p. 1130; F. Charatan, 'Dozens of patients allege unnecessary heart surgery', *BMJ*, vol. 326, May 2003, p. 1055; J. Lenzer, 'Health care group agrees $500m settlement for unnecessary surgery', *BMJ*, vol. 333, Jul. 2006, p. 59.

22   J. Lenzer, 'Health care group agrees $500m', *BMJ*, vol. 333, Jul. 2006, p. 59.

23   R. Moynihan, 'Another US health care giant is hit by scandal', *BMJ*, vol. 327, Nov. 2003, p. 1128.

Chapter 10

1   J. Groopman, *How Doctors Think*, Scribe, Melbourne, 2007.

2   R.M. Epstein, B.S. Alper and T.E. Quill, 'Communicating evidence for participatory decision making', *Journal of the American Medical Association*, vol. 291, May 2004, pp. 2359–66.

3   J. Harrington, L.M. Noble and S.P. Newman, 'Improving patients' communication with doctors: A systematic review of intervention studies', *Patient Education and Counseling*, vol. 52, Jan. 2004, pp. 7–16.

4   National Health and Medical Research Council, 'Making decisions about tests and treatments: Principles for better communication between health care consumers and health care professionals', Australian Government, Canberra, 2006.

5   Groopman, *How Doctors Think*, p. 76.

6   Epstein, Alper and Quill, 'Communicating evidence', pp. 2359–66.

7   Interview with Dr Christine Connors, 2007.

8   J.E. Jordan and R.H. Osborne, 'Chronic disease self-management education programs: Challenges ahead', *Medical Journal of Australia*, vol. 186, pp. 84–7.

9   M. Sweet, *The Big Fat Conspiracy: How to protect your family's health*, ABC Books, Sydney, 2007.

Conclusion

1   See, for example, J. Clayton et al., 'Asking questions can help: Development and preliminary evaluation of a question prompt list for palliantive care patients', *British Journal of Cancer*, vol. 89, Dec. 2003, pp. 2069–77; P. Kinnersley et al., 'Interventions before consultations for helping patients address their information needs', *Cochrane Database of Systematic Reviews*, 2007.

Acknowledgements

A big thankyou to Chris Coulter, one of Ray's oldest friends, who claims, somewhat plausibly, that the title for the book emerged from his lips during a conversation the pair had at Coogee, in Sydney. Whether this is true or not, Chris has considered Melissa and Ray to be his ghost writers ever since. Rebecca Kaiser, at Allen & Unwin, was her warm, charming, efficient and encouraging self throughout.

Thanks to the following people, who commented on drafts or extracts from the book and whose feedback was extremely helpful: Professor Rachelle Buchbinder, Department of Epidemiology and Preventative Medicine, Monash University; Sir Iain Chalmers, Editor, James Lind Library; Taddy Dickersin, Professor, Department of Epidemiology, Johns Hopkins Bloomberg School of Public Health; Simon Chapman, Professor of Public Health, University of Sydney; David Henry, CEO, Institute for Clinical Evaluative Sciences, Toronto; Libby Roughead, Associate Professor, University of South Australia;

Hubert van Griensven, Consultant Physiotherapist, Southend University Hospital NHS Foundation Trust, in the United Kingdom; Merrilyn Walton, Associate Professor of Patient Safety, University of Sydney.

Particular thanks go to Les Marshall, a pensioner from Gatton in rural Queensland, who volunteered to be our 'guinea pig', reading the draft manuscript from the perspective of an older person with a chronic disease. We were enormously reassured by his feedback: 'Everyone should read this book,' he told us.

Melissa would also like to acknowledge Les Irwig, Judy Irwig and Lyndal Trevena, her co-authors on *Smart Health Choices*, a book that also aims to empower people to become better informed when making health decisions.

The original concept for this book came from Ray Moynihan, who drafted chapters 1, 2, 3, 7, 9. Melissa Sweet drafted chapters 4, 5, 6, 8 and 10.

Index